MW00782595

IVF SUCCESS

An Evidence-Based Guide to
Getting Pregnant and Clues to Why
You Are Not Pregnant Now

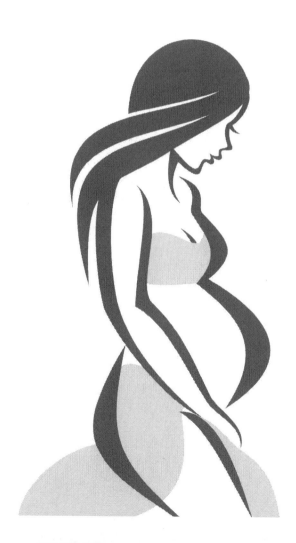

Praise for *"IVF Success"*

"Reading this book helped to reassure me that my fertility specialist was on the right track because the reasoning behind each protocol was in the book. There were definitely some suggestions that I will be discussing with my fertility specialist now that I am aware of other strategies. The book helped me to gain a greater understanding of my failed IVF."

Kellie-Marie Gaskell
Primary School Teacher
Melbourne, Australia

"This book is truly a gem. It is easy to read, clear, and concise, yet covers all the essentials and critical facts for couples to appreciate why they should seek fertility treatments early, understand the limitations, and not be lured into accepting unproven treatments.

Every Assisted Reproductive Center and IVF patient support group around the world should have this book available to their patients, clients, and members.

Most importantly, this is a 'must read' for fertility specialists to bring us down to earth and stay true to our mission to do no harm and practice sound evidence-based medicine."

Dr. Suresh Nair
IVF Specialist
Singapore

"I would have loved this book before I started infertility treatment! I would give it 10 out of 10. It is almost like an IVF handbook; everyone should get a copy before they start."

Wendy Keating
Primary School Teacher
Melbourne, Australia

"As an IVF specialist, Raphael Kuhn ensured his patients received a holistic approach to their physical and emotional well-being. This book is an extension of his practice philosophy as he aims to demystify the sometimes confusing world of Assisted Reproductive Technology and simply explain all the different treatments available to patients these days, so they can be active and informed participants in their treatment."

Marianne Tome
Counselling Manager
Melbourne IVF
Australia

"Based on years of experience and backed by extensive research, this book is essential reading for anyone whose IVF treatment has been unsuccessful."

Juliet Robinson
Chairperson Melbourne IVF Human
Research and Ethics Committee
Australia

"This book is easy to read and easy to understand. Reading this book has informed me of the things I need to do in order to have a successful IVF pregnancy. It has outstanding information about different conditions and procedures that can be helpful to many couples and singles."

Erin Azzopardi
Medical Nutritionist
Melbourne, Australia

"This book will be a useful, comprehensive resource for those considering IVF treatment. It will help them understand why they may have experienced difficulties conceiving and provide a basis for exploring these with their fertility specialist.

It is reassuring that the information provided is factual and evidence-based, rather than just opinions."

Sandra Dill AM
CEO ACCESS
Australia's National Infertility Network

"When you turn to IVF for help, you don't want fluff. You want cold, hard facts. The style of this book is fantastic."

Vivienne Payne,
Melbourne, Australia

"This book is an ideal, very readable, factual guide to achieving the best possible outcome from your IVF treatment."

Dr. Koen Geerinckx
IVF Specialist
Belgium

IVF SUCCESS

An Evidence-Based Guide to Getting Pregnant and Clues to Why You Are Not Pregnant Now

DR RAPHAEL KUHN

MB BS (Melb) FRCOG FRANZCOG

Published in Australia by
ISO Media
Address: PO Box 1126 Hawksburn, Victoria 3142 Australia
Email: raph@raphaelkuhn.com
Website: www.raphaelkuhn.com

First published in Australia 2017
Copyright © Raphael Kuhn 2017

All rights reserved. No part of this publication may be reproduced, stored in a retrieval system, or transmitted, in any form or by any means without the prior written permission of the publisher, nor be otherwise circulated in any form of binding or cover other than that in which it is published and without a similar condition being imposed on the subsequent purchaser.

National Library of Australia Cataloguing-in-Publication entry

Creator: Kuhn, Raphael, author.
Title: IVF success: An Evidence-Based Guide to Getting Pregnant
          and Clues to Why You Are Not Pregnant Now / Raphael Kuhn.
ISBN: 978-0-6480353-2-9 (Createspace paperback)
ISBN: 978-0-6480353-1-2 (ebook)
Subjects: Fertilization in vitro, Human--Australia.
          Evidence-based medicine--Australia.
          Pregnancy--Australia.

Cover design by Nelly Murariu, PixBee Design
Book formatting by Nelly Murariu, PixBee Design
Printed by Createspace

Disclaimer
All care has been taken in the preparation of the information herein, but no responsibility can be accepted by the publisher or author for any damages resulting from the misinterpretation of this work. All contact details given in this book were current at the time of publication but are subject to change.

The advice given in this book is based on the experience of the individuals described. Professionals should be consulted for individual problems. The author and publisher shall not be responsible for any person with regard to any loss or damage caused directly or indirectly by the information in this book.

This book is dedicated to
Ian Johnston AM,
'Father of IVF in Australia,'
and those who have yet to
achieve their goal.

CONTENTS

Introduction

Some describe IVF treatment as miraculous. It can bring you immeasurable happiness in the form of a perfect bundle of joy, but it can also be responsible for profound disappointment and sadness when it does not go as planned. The emotional and financial costs of undergoing IVF are considerable, especially when you have to undergo multiple cycles, which are physically and psychologically exhausting, not to mention expensive. Each time you begin with a rush of hope, and when that hope is dashed yet again, it can make you feel desperate.

This desperation when things are not working out makes you vulnerable and more willing to try anything that might help, even when there is no proof that it will. Unfortunately, there are many people willing to take advantage of your deepest desires by offering these ineffective services. For example, there is currently no good high quality evidence that IVF outcomes are improved by the treatment of uterine Natural Killer cells, yet a very large number of patients turn to this after experiencing unsuccessful outcomes.

I have written this book in the hope of spreading evidence-based information, so that you are fully aware of the facts and fiction surrounding IVF treatment and have the best chance at IVF success.

I began my career as a specialist obstetrician and gynecologist, then focused on endoscopic (keyhole) surgery, and finally spent more than 15 years as an IVF specialist. This was followed by two years of providing independent second opinions to unsuccessful IVF patients. It was that experience that prompted me to write this book.

While providing these second opinions, it became apparent that there were major problems: incomplete information, communication breakdowns, misunderstandings, and unrealistic expectations. There was also a desperate desire to believe that unproven treatments might work, many adopting the attitude that if a treatment causes no harm, they might as well give it a try since they have nothing to lose. However, there is an emotional and a financial cost when these "harmless" practices do not work.

Let's take a look at some of the facts presented in this book:

Q The age of the female IVF patient (whose eggs are used for fertilization whether using one's own eggs or those of a donor) is the most important factor determining the outcome of IVF treatment. It does not matter how young you look, there is nothing that can change your age or the age of your eggs. Age is going to be a major factor in infertility until we learn to populate older ovaries with young eggs derived from stem cells. As you age, more of your eggs are chromosomally abnormal, and therefore, result in the creation of abnormal embryos. Also, as you get older, your ovarian reserve, your capacity to produce fertilizable eggs, goes down.

Q It is tempting to want to rush into treatment, but if you took the time to address lifestyle issues, including weight, you could save yourself a lot of heartache and money, and you may not even need IVF.

Q There are many ways in which your ovaries can be stimulated to produce more fertilizable eggs, so that hopefully, more embryos are created. However, more may not always be better, and increasing the dose of ovulatory stimulant may not be the answer.

Q Good embryo transfer technique is critical for the best possible chance of a favorable outcome. Trauma, which may result in bleeding (blood is toxic to embryos) or uterine contractions (which could expel the embryo after transfer), must be avoided if at all possible.

Q A straightforward technique, endometrial scratching, that can be performed as an office procedure, may significantly improve the likelihood of success if recurrent implantation failure is the problem.

Q There is a simple blood test, serum progesterone, available that can predict the likelihood of an unfavorable endometrium (uterine lining) for embryo implantation in a stimulated cycle (one in which eggs are collected). Therefore, it would seem unwise to perform a fresh embryo transfer in a cycle that is predicted to have an unfavorable endometrium. In this case, it is wiser to freeze all embryos and individually thaw and transfer them in subsequent natural or artificial menstrual cycles until a pregnancy is achieved.

There are many more areas of interest and relevance covered in this book. If your IVF treatment has been unsuccessful thus far, I hope that you not only find some answers in this book, but also learn things that enable you to have a more engaging and informed consultation with your fertility specialist.

The earlier chapters discuss issues that may be very relevant to you, including age, weight, lifestyle, uterine fibroids, uterine lining, endometriosis, and the immune system. Subsequent chapters address topics that include IVF stimulation protocols, problems with fertilization, embryo transfer technique, and luteal phase support. The final chapters, entitled "What Next?," raise topics for discussion and consideration with your fertility specialist.

This should lead to a clear plan of action that best suits your circumstances. One size does not fit all.

While there is some technical language, anyone who is currently going through IVF treatment, or who has gone through it in the past, will be familiar with most of these terms. There is also a glossary at the end of the book for your reference.

CHAPTER 1

Is It My Age?

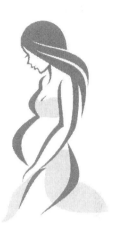

The Perfect Couple

Jane was 38 when she met Michael, who was 42 at the time. The timing was perfect: neither had been in a recent long term relationship, and both wanted to find a life partner, settle down, and have a family. Their successful careers ensured their financial security, and they seemed ideally matched, sharing a surprisingly large number of common interests. Six months later, they were married and on their honeymoon.

The Problem

Despite a regular menstrual cycle and frequent lovemaking, six months later, Jane was still not pregnant. They consulted their proactive family physician (general practitioner), who felt that, due to their ages, there was no time to waste, especially since they wanted to have at least two children. He referred them to a fertility specialist.

A blood test showed that Jane was ovulating, and Michael's sperm test was normal. Jane had an ultrasound examination that confirmed both of her fallopian tubes were open; it also showed no evidence of severe endometriosis, ovarian pathology, or uterine fibroids that might interfere with embryo implantation. They decided against having a laparoscopy to exclude mild endometriosis since Jane had no symptoms suggesting the condition.

Their problem appeared to be one of unexplained infertility.

After an in-depth discussion with their fertility specialist, they decided that IVF was their best treatment option.

First Stimulated IVF Cycle

Jane and Michael's first IVF treatment cycle was an antagonist cycle. Jane's ovaries were stimulated with daily Follicle Stimulating Hormone (FSH) injections. Premature release of eggs was prevented with daily Gonadotrophin Releasing Hormone (GnRH) antagonist injections, which were started once the follicles had begun active growth. Final egg ripening was achieved with a trigger injection of human Chorionic Gonadotrophin (hCG) 36 hours before egg collection.

They felt this treatment was easy to follow, and the results were not very different from those of other protocols (hormonal drug combinations) that could be used to stimulate Jane's ovaries to produce a good number of eggs for collection.

Before starting, Jane had her ovarian reserve evaluated; in other words, a blood test was carried out to measure the capacity of her ovaries to produce eggs that could be fertilized. It was at the lower limit of normal, which suggested that her response to ovarian stimulation using a standard dose of FSH might not be ideal, so a higher dose was used.

Eleven eggs were collected, eight of which were fertilizable (mature). Six fertilized, four normally. The embryos were then grown to day five (blastocyst stage) with two making the distance. One was transferred fresh, and the other was frozen for later use.

Ten days after the fresh embryo transfer, a blood test revealed a detectable, but low, level of hCG (pregnancy hormone). The low level indicated that it was not an ongoing pregnancy. Two days later, Jane was bleeding.

First Thaw Cycle

With the onset of Jane's next natural menstrual period, they embarked on a thawed embryo transfer cycle. Five days after ovulation, their frozen day five embryo was thawed and transferred.

Jane's period arrived two days before her pregnancy blood test was due to be performed. When the test was done, there was no detectable pregnancy hormone. Jane and Michael saw both their fertility specialist and their IVF counsellor to help them deal with their disappointment. This is unsurprising for anyone who has put in so much effort and has not had a good outcome.

They decided to persevere and continue with their IVF treatment.

Second Stimulated IVF Cycle

Two months later, Jane and Michael started their next stimulated IVF cycle.

This time they used Pre-implantation Genetic Screening (PGS), which involved doing a biopsy (taking some cells) of each embryo that grew to day five. The cells were then tested to see if the embryo was euploid (chromosomally normal) or aneuploid (chromosomally abnormal).

They also used a different stimulation protocol (a variation on the hormone injections they had used in their first stimulated cycle). The dose of FSH was increased in the hope of increasing the number of eggs collected, which in turn, would hopefully increase the number of embryos suitable for biopsy.

Fourteen eggs were collected. Ten were mature, and seven fertilized normally. Three grew to day five and were biopsied and frozen, awaiting the results of genetic testing. One proved to be chromosomally normal.

Second Thaw Cycle

The chromosomally normal embryo was thawed and transferred in a subsequent natural cycle that resulted in an ongoing singleton intrauterine pregnancy.

Elizabeth was born last December.

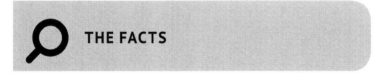

THE FACTS

Your age is the most important factor determining your chance of having a child through IVF. There are two main reasons for this:

Firstly, there is an ever-increasing proportion of chromosomally abnormal eggs (which would result in chromosomally abnormal embryos) after 30 years of age.

In 2014, an exceptionally informative study examined the relationship between the age of the female partner and the number and type of chromosomal abnormalities in more than 15,000 embryos.[1]

Age of female partner	Percentage of chromosomally abnormal embryos
30 years	31.0%
37 years	42.6%
40 years	58.2%
42 years	75.1%
44 years	88.2%
>44 years	100%

Franasiak JM et al. Fertil. Steril. 2014; 101:656-663.

On a positive note, the ongoing pregnancy rate is the same when a chromosomally normal embryo is transferred, irrespective of the age of the woman from whom the egg was collected. In other words, your age does not matter as long as a chromosomally normal embryo is transferred.

However, the transfer of a chromosomally normal embryo is not a guarantee of an ongoing pregnancy or delivery of a normal, healthy baby because it does not exclude the possibility of other genetic disorders or the development of anatomical abnormalities.

Chromosomally abnormal embryos may fail to implant, yield a positive pregnancy test but not an ongoing pregnancy, or end in miscarriage. They will never result in the birth of a normal, healthy baby.

---

1   Franasiak JM, Forman EJ, Hong KH, Werner MD, Upham KM, Treff NR, and Scott RT. *The nature of aneuploidy with increasing age of the female partner: a review of 15,169 consecutive trophectoderm biopsies evaluated with comprehensive chromosomal screening.* Fertil. Steril. 2014; 101:656-663.

Secondly, there is a decline in ovarian reserve (the capacity of the ovary to produce eggs capable of fertilization) with increasing age because the pool of follicles containing immature eggs is depleted during the reproductive years.

The best markers of ovarian reserve are Anti-Mullerian Hormone (AMH) and Antral Follicle Count (AFC).

Anti-Mullerian Hormone (AMH)

AMH is produced by the cells that line follicles awaiting further development. It is believed that AMH levels are the first marker of ovarian reserve to diminish with age, so they may be an early sign of a diminished ovarian reserve.

The predictive value of very low AMH <0.6 ng/ml (<4.3pmol/L) was reported in 2016 for over 5,000 IVF cycles.[2] The cancellation rate was 54%, and the live birth rate was 9.5%. This meant that more than half of the women with very low levels of AMH had their cycle cancelled, and less than one in ten successfully had a baby.

There are several factors that can affect AMH results:

Q AMH results may differ for the same blood sample when measured by different laboratories because of the assay (test) used.

Q The way the blood sample is handled can also have an effect (e.g. using inappropriate blood collection tubes or mailing samples before they are centrifuged (spun down) can cause problems with testing).

---

2   Seler DB, Tal O, Wantman E, Edul P, and Baker VL. *Prognostic indicators of assisted reproduction technology outcomes of cycles with ultralow serum antimullerian hormone: a multivariate analysis of over 5000 autologous cycles from the Society for Assisted Reproductive Technology Clinic Outcome Reporting System database for 2012-2013.* Fertil. Steril. 2016; 105:385-393.

Q AMH levels may be falsely elevated (by up to 40% at room temperature) if the sample is not centrifuged immediately.

Q Taking the oral contraceptive pill can impact AMH results. Levels may be at least 20% lower while on the pill than they would be if the test is repeated once the pill has been ceased for three months.

Q The belief that AMH levels do not vary during the menstrual cycle has been brought into question by a very recent study.[3] One in three women with low AMH levels and two out of three women with reduced AMH levels were reclassified because of the significant variation observed in AMH levels during the menstrual cycle (i.e. a significantly large number were told they had a reduced ovarian reserve when they actually did not).

It is clear that clinical decisions should not be made on a single AMH measurement but should form part of an overall assessment, including the following:

Antral Follicle Count (AFC)

AFC is defined as the number of follicles (two to nine millimeters in diameter) visible when a transvaginal ultrasound examination is conducted on days one to five of the menstrual cycle. However, a study in 2011 showed that the AFC predictive value remains

3   Hadlow N, Brown SJ, Habib A, Wardrop R, Joseph J, Gillett M, McGuire R, and Conradie J. *Quantifying the intraindividual variation of antimullerian hormone in the ovarian cycle.* Fertil. Steril. 2016; 106:1230-1237.

unchanged across the menstrual cycle (i.e. this measurement does not need to be confined to the first five days of the cycle).[4]

While an AFC of 14 or more follicles is indicative of a normal ovarian reserve, an AFC of less than seven is considered to reflect a reduced ovarian reserve, and an AFC of less than four indicates a severely reduced reserve.

Other Markers of Ovarian Reserve

Another marker of ovarian reserve is the basal serum Follicle Stimulating Hormone (FSH) level, which is usually measured on day two or three of the menstrual cycle, but can be done as late as day five. An elevated FSH level indicates a depleted pool of follicles and a decreased likelihood of ovarian response to stimulation. It should be noted that elevated basal serum FSH is one of the later signs of reduced ovarian reserve.

A FSH level between 5 and 10 I.U./L is considered normal, between 10 and 15 I.U./L borderline, and greater than 15 I.U./L elevated and indicative of increased likelihood of stimulation failure.

If basal FSH is part of treatment planning, the highest reported level should be used to determine treatment. Subsequent lower levels do not correlate with better outcomes (i.e. there is no value in waiting for a cycle with a lower basal FSH level to start stimulation).

A basal serum estradiol level greater than 80pg/ml (294pmol/L) has also been shown to correlate with lower pregnancy rates, even if basal FSH is normal.

---

4   Rombauts L, Onwude JL, Chew HW, and Vollenhoven B. *The predictive value of antral follicle count remains unchanged across the menstrual cycle.* Fertil. Steril. 2011; 96:1514-1518.

Therefore, basal FSH and estradiol should be measured together. When both are elevated, the response to stimulation is very poor.

There was a study published in 2011, entitled "Association between number of eggs collected and live birth in IVF treatment: analysis of 400,135 treatment cycles."[5] The paper contained a nomogram (table) that made it possible to easily calculate the chance of live birth based on age and the number of eggs collected.

Fig 1.1: Nomogram to calculate predicted probability of live birth based on age and number of eggs collected.

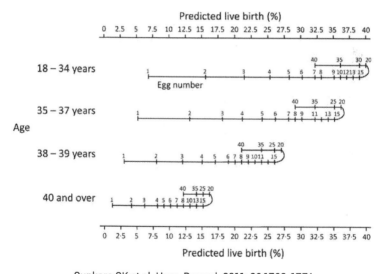

Sunkara SK et al. Hum. Reprod. 2011; 26:1768-1774.

5   Sunkara SK, Rittenberg V, Raine-Fenning N, Bhattacharya S, Zamora J, and Coomarasamy A. *Association between the number of eggs and live birth in IVF treatment: an analysis of 400,135 treatment cycles.* Hum. Reprod. 2011; 26:1768-1774.

Age of Male Partner

Men's age also has an impact on IVF outcomes.

A study evaluating nearly 2,000 couples having IVF because of tubal disease found that the male partners who were more than 39 years old were less likely than younger men to have a good outcome.[6]

Another report analysing 237 donor egg cycles identified a decline in both pregnancy and live birth rates with increasing age of the male.[7]

There is an increased risk of autism spectrum and psychiatric disorders in offspring with increasing paternal age.[8]

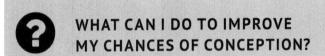

WHAT CAN I DO TO IMPROVE MY CHANCES OF CONCEPTION?

There is no doubt that age is the most important factor determining the chance of having an IVF baby; this is due to the declining ovarian reserve, combined with the ever-increasing proportion of chromosomally abnormal eggs as a woman ages.

The nomogram (table) mentioned above, showing the correlation of age with the number of eggs collected and the live birth rate,

6   de la Rochebrochard E, de Mouzon J, Thepot F, Thonneau P. *Fathers over 40 and increased failure to conceive :the lessons of in vitro fertilization in France.* Fertil. Steril. 2006; 85:1420-1424.
7   Robertshaw I, Khoury J, Abdallah ME, Wankoo P, and Hofmann GE. *The effect of paternal age on outcome in assisted reproductive technology using the ovum donation model.* Reprod. Sci. 2014; 21:590-593.
8   D'Onofrio BM, Rickert ME, Frans E, Kuja-Halkola R, Almoqvist C, Sjolander A, Larrson H and Lichtenstein P. *Paternal age at childbearing and offspring psychiatric and academic morbidity.* JAMA Psychiatry 2014; 71:432-438.

provides a very helpful guide to the likelihood of success at different ages.

While you cannot change your age, an optimal Body Mass Index (BMI) and healthy lifestyle (see Chapters 2 and 3) will maximize your chances of conception.

CHAPTER 2

Is It My Weight?

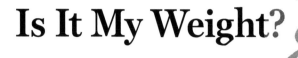

The Young Couple

Tanya was 28 years old. She had her facial hair and acne, which are commonly associated with Polycystic Ovarian Syndrome (PCOS), under control but not her weight. Her infrequent periods made it difficult to predict or confirm when she was ovulating. Despite frequent intercourse with her partner, Nick, there were countless negative urinary pregnancy tests over eight months.

Standing 5'3"(160 cm.) tall and weighing 176 lbs. (80 kg.), Tanya had a Body Mass Index (BMI) of 31. An ultrasound examination performed vaginally revealed polycystic ovaries (ovaries with lots of little cysts), but no other abnormality. Their family physician (general practitioner) arranged for Nick to have a sperm test. The result was normal.

They were then referred to a fertility specialist.

First Line Treatment

Neither clomiphene alone, nor a combination of clomiphene and metformin (pills used alone or together to induce ovulation), was successful in providing Tanya with a regular cycle in which ovulation occurred. Daily injections of Follicle Stimulating Hormone (FSH) were tried and monitored with ultrasound scans.

Despite slowly and carefully increasing the dose of FSH, Tanya always overshot and made too many follicles. This made both timed intercourse and intrauterine Insemination (IUI) unsafe treatments because of the high risk of multiple pregnancy (twins or more).

The Next Step

Tanya and Nick's patience ran out, and they decided to proceed with IVF. This offered them a more controllable treatment option.

A single embryo could be transferred fresh, and any surplus good quality embryos frozen. Alternatively, all embryos could be frozen if there was a significant risk of OHSS (Ovarian Hyperstimulation Syndrome). OHSS is an ovarian stimulation complication in which too many follicles develop, and it can cause excessive fluid retention that may require hospitalization. Tanya was at risk because she had PCOS.

Pre-implantation Genetic Screening (testing cells from each embryo to see if the embryos were chromosomally normal) was discussed, but Tanya and Nick decided against it, both because of the additional cost involved and because Tanya's young age made it very likely that good numbers of chromosomally normal embryos would be created.

A Gonadotrophin Releasing Hormone (GnRH) antagonist cycle was started. This involved daily injections of FSH, accompanied by daily injections of GnRH antagonist once follicles started growing actively. The GnRH antagonist prevented premature release of eggs before they were ready for collection. A lower dose of daily FSH injections than usual was used to minimize the risk of OHSS. This type of stimulation cycle also provided the option of triggering (ripening the eggs for collection) with a

GnRH agonist, eliminating the risk of severe OHSS associated with a hCG trigger if a very large number of follicles developed.

Fourteen good-sized follicles developed, and twelve eggs were collected, eight of which were mature (fertilizable). Six fertilized normally, but only one continued growing to day five. This embryo was transferred fresh.

Ten days later, Tanya and Nick were thrilled to learn that Tanya was pregnant and her pregnancy hormone levels were very good. Their joy, however, was short-lived. Tanya started bleeding, the bleeding got heavier, and she miscarried.

What next?

Having come to terms with their pregnancy loss, Tanya and Nick asked their fertility specialist if there was anything they could do to improve their chances the next time around. Their fertility specialist explained that if Tanya reduced her Body Mass Index (BMI) by losing weight, she would not only increase the chances of conceiving, but also reduce the risk of miscarriage and other pregnancy complications.

Tanya joined a structured and monitored weight reduction program and started a moderate half-hour daily exercise program. Six months later, she was 134 lbs. (62kg.), with a normal BMI of 24, and she had a regular 30-day menstrual cycle.

She conceived naturally two months later and is due later this year.

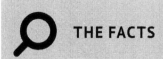

THE FACTS

Body Mass Index (BMI) is an important measurement relating to weight and height. It is calculated by dividing a person's weight in pounds (lbs) by their height in inches squared (in^2) multiplied by 703 or by simply dividing their weight in kilograms (kg) by their height in meters squared (m^2).

Commonly accepted BMI ranges are:
- Q Underweight − under 18.5
- Q Normal − 18.5 to 25
- Q Overweight − 25 to 30
- Q Obese − over 30

It has been well known for some time that obesity has a significant adverse effect on pregnancy, causing problems such as pregnancy-induced hypertension (high blood pressure), gestational diabetes, thromboembolism, fetal macrosomia (very large baby), and unexplained stillbirth. Obesity is also linked with an increased rate of Caesarean sections and post-operative wound infections, as well as an increased risk of miscarriage.

It is only in the last decade that closer attention has been paid to obesity (BMI > 30), being overweight (BMI > 25 but < 30), and their impact on IVF treatment and outcomes. Obesity is a high oxidative stress (cell damaging) state associated with an increased likelihood of failure to achieve a live birth.[1]

---

1   Luke B, Brown MB, Missmer SA, Bukulmez O, Leach R, and Stern JE. *The effect of increasing obesity on the response to and outcome of assisted reproductive technology: a national survey.* Fertil. Steril. 2011;96:820-825.

There have been several comprehensive reviews of the subject. An analysis of 33 studies reviewing the outcomes of over 47,967 IVF treatment cycles concluded that women who were overweight or obese had lower clinical pregnancy rates, higher miscarriage rates, and lower live birth rates than women with a normal BMI.[2]

In 2013, at the European Society of Human Reproduction and Embryology (ESHRE) meeting in London, El-Toukly presented a paper on obesity and IVF outcomes, based on more than 6,500 treatment cycles.

There was a statically significant result (hard evidence) showing that a lower number of eggs was collected when a woman's BMI was 30 or over. Statistically significantly lower clinical pregnancy rates and live birth rates were observed if her BMI was over 25. The same applied to miscarriage rates, which were statistically significantly higher if her BMI was greater than 25.

Being underweight (BMI under 18.5) can also cause problems. It can lead to secondary amenorrhoea (periods stopping for more than six months) and is associated with an increased risk of miscarriage. It can also lead to a compromised response to ovarian stimulation in Ovulation Induction (OI), Intrauterine Insemination (IUI), and IVF treatment cycles.

---

2   Rittenberg V, Seshadri S, Sunkara SK, Sobaleva S, Oteng-Ntim E, and El-Toukhy T. *Effect of body mass index on IVF treatment outcome: an updated systematic review and meta-analysis.* Reprod. Biomed. Online 2011:23:421-439.

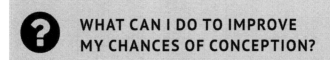

WHAT CAN I DO TO IMPROVE MY CHANCES OF CONCEPTION?

Obesity, or even just being overweight, is associated with a lower number of eggs being collected, lower clinical pregnancy rates, lower live birth rates, and higher rates of miscarriage.

Being underweight can also lead to problems.

Maintaining a healthy weight is a concrete step you can take to help attain IVF success.

An optimal BMI (between 18.5 and 25) significantly improves your chances of conceiving, both naturally and with IVF.

CHAPTER 3

Is It My Lifestyle?

Generation X

Sally, who was 36, and her husband, Sam, who was 37, were desperate to start a family. An unexpected inheritance had paid off their mortgage. They tried very hard for six months to get pregnant and were becoming increasingly stressed, especially Sally.

Sally dealt with her stress by talking to her extensive network of girlfriends over multiple cups of coffee and a cigarette or two, and relaxing with her husband over a couple of glasses of white wine in the evenings. More often than not, they finished the bottle. Sally also tried to cope with her stress by engaging in regular, almost daily, intense gym sessions.

Sam got support from his friends over a few beers on weekends. They joked that there might be a problem with his "swimmers." As it turns out, there was.

Sam's family physician (general practitioner) arranged for him to have a sperm test. This revealed not only a low sperm count, but also a high percentage of abnormal sperm. The test was repeated, and the result was the same.

Sally and Sam were referred to a fertility specialist.

Sound Advice

Their fertility specialist insisted on lifestyle changes because alcohol, nicotine, and excessive caffeine intake and exercise are all known to adversely affect chances of both natural and IVF conception.

Sally stopped smoking and drinking, reduced her caffeine intake, and moderated her exercise schedule. Sam stopped drinking as well.

Their fertility specialist did, however, reassure them that stress, whether related to their treatment or other factors, would not adversely affect the outcome.

It took them three months to get into good shape. Sam had another sperm test, but it was still significantly abnormal.

Their first stimulated IVF treatment cycle resulted in a singleton intrauterine pregnancy with a readily detectable, normal fetal heart rate confirmed by ultrasound.

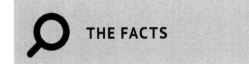

THE FACTS

Stress

Stress does not affect IVF treatment outcome. A systematic review and meta-analysis of 14 prospective psychosocial studies, involving a total of 3,583 infertile women undergoing IVF treatment, concluded, "The findings of this meta-analysis should reassure women and doctors that emotional distress caused by infertility problems or other events co-occurring with treatment will not compromise the chances of becoming pregnant."[1]

Distress, however, can mean that patients stop treatment prematurely, before the optimal number of cycles to get pregnant has been completed. It is therefore important to address any issues early and get support, including from your IVF counselor, to assist you in continuing treatment for the optimal period of time.

Exercise

Sensible exercise improves results of IVF treatment. Moderate exercise in the female who is the source of eggs is associated with improved IVF outcomes.[2] However, vigorous exercise is correlated with reduced IVF success.[3, 4] While engaging in very vigorous exercise is discouraged, 30 minutes of moderate aerobic exercise per day would be endorsed by most fertility specialists.

Alcohol

Do not drink alcohol if you are planning to get pregnant.

In a study involving 2,574 couples entitled "Effect of Alcohol Consumption on IVF," women who consumed four or more drinks per week had a 16% lower chance of having a live birth than

1   Bolvin J, Griffiths E, and Venetis CA. *Emotional distress in infertile women and failure and failure of assisted reproductive technologies: meta-analysis of prospective psycho-social studies.* BMJ 2011; 342
2   Evenson KR, Calhoun AC, Herring AH, Pritchard D, Wen F, and Steiner AZ. *Association of physical activity in the past year and immediately after in vitro fertilization on pregnancy.* Fertil. Steril. 2014; 101:1047-1054.
3   Gudmundsdottir SL, Flanders WD, and Augestad LB. *Physical activity and fertility in women: the North Trendelag Health Study.* Hum. Reprod. 2009; 24:3196-3204.
4   Wise LA, Rothman KJ, Mikkelsen EM, Sorensen HT, Riis AH, and Hatch EE. *A prospective cohort study of physical activity and time to pregnancy.* Fertil. Steril. 2012; 97:1136-1142.

those who drank less.[5] The live birth rate was 21% lower among couples who both drank four or more drinks per week, compared with those who drank less.

While weekly white wine consumption by men increased the likelihood of poor sperm morphology (physical form) by 43%, red wine consumption at the same frequency was associated with a 23% higher occurrence of poor sperm concentration (count).

Smoking

Smoking has a very negative impact on the success of IVF treatment.

A report involving all IVF clinics in the Netherlands studied the smoking habits of 8,457 women. It summed up its findings with this statement: "Our study found that the effect of smoking more than one cigarette per day for a year reduced a woman's chances of having a live birth through IVF by 28%—that's the same percentage disadvantage that occurs between a 20 year old woman and a 30 year old woman."[6]

It went on to state, "Smoking has the greatest effect on women with unexplained infertility problems. In these patients, IVF treatment led to 20.7% of non-smokers achieving a live birth, compared with 13.4% of smokers. These results indicate that smoking may actually be causing the problems these women are experiencing."

---

5   Rossi BV, Berry KF, Hornstein MD, Cramer DW, Ehrlich S, and Missmer SA. *Effect of Alcohol Consumption on In Vitro Fertilization.* Obstet. Gynecol. 2011; 117[1]: 136-142.
6   Lintsen AME, Pasker-de Jong PCM, de Boer EJ, Burger CW, Jansen CAM, Braat DDM, and van Leeuwen FE. *Effects of subfertility cause smoking and bodt weight on success rate of IVF.* Hum. Reprod .2005; 20:1867-1875.

A subsequent review of the available literature confirmed the conclusions of the Dutch study.[7]

There is research to indicate that a number of substances found in tobacco products, including nicotine and its breakdown products, not only affect follicular development (growth of follicles) and egg maturation (ripening), but also uterine receptivity (favorability of uterine lining for embryo implantation).

Caffeine

You should limit your daily caffeine intake because excessive consumption may compromise the results of IVF treatment.

A 2012 Danish study involving 3,959 women found that drinking five or more cups of coffee per day reduced the clinical pregnancy rate of IVF treatment cycles by half. The live birth rate may be reduced by up to 40%, compared with those who drank less.[8]

---

7   Waylen AL, Metwally M, Jones GL, Wilkinson AJ, and Ledger WL. *Effects of cigarette smoking upon clinical outcomes of assisted reproduction: a meta-analysis.* Hum. Reprod. Update 2009; 15:31-44.
8   Kesmodel US. *Coffee and IVF.* Annual Meeting of European Society of Human Reproduction and Embryology, 2012: Abstract O-202.

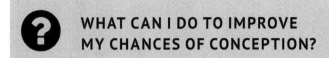

WHAT CAN I DO TO IMPROVE MY CHANCES OF CONCEPTION?

While stress reduction will help you to cope with IVF treatment, stress itself will not compromise the outcome.

Smoking increases the likelihood of IVF treatment failure, as does alcohol, excessive coffee consumption, and excessive exercise.

A healthy lifestyle significantly improves your pregnancy prospects.

CHAPTER 4

Is It My Uterus?

Correct Treatment But...

Kate was 36 years and had never been pregnant. She and her partner Peter, who was 34, were informed that the most likely explanation for their year of primary infertility was Peter's sperm quality.

He had had three sperm tests, and all revealed more than 96% abnormal forms, which are either unable to attach to an egg or to penetrate the egg's shell (zona pellucida). IVF with ICSI, Intra-Cytoplasmic Sperm Injection (injecting a single sperm into a single egg), was recommended.

No contributory factor had been identified in Kate, although it was noted on a recent ultrasound examination performed by a general radiology department that she had several intramural (within the uterine wall) and subserosal (on the surface of the uterus) fibroids that were two centimeters in diameter.

Their first stimulated IVF cycle resulted in the creation of three very good quality day five embryos (blastocysts). One embryo was transferred fresh, and the other two were frozen. A positive pregnancy test resulted, but the pregnancy did not last.

Why It Wasn't Successful

Kate and Peter were understandably very disappointed, and their fertility specialist was surprised because the quality of the embryo was outstanding and the embryo transfer had been very smooth and without trauma. They discussed the possibility of some factor interfering with implantation.

An ultrasound examination was performed by a gynecological ultrasound subspecialist via the vagina, with an injection of contrast medium to clearly outline the uterine cavity. A two-centimeter submucosal (under the lining of the uterus) fibroid was identified, and more than 50% of it was protruding into the uterine cavity. It was hysteroscopically (through the vagina and via the cervical canal) removed in conjunction with an endometrial (uterine lining) biopsy, which revealed no evidence of endometritis (inflammation of the uterine lining).

A thawed embryo transfer in a natural cycle three months later resulted in a successful pregnancy.

Harry was delivered normally and close to full-term.

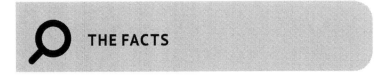

THE FACTS

Uterine fibroids are the most common benign (non-cancerous) tumor in women of reproductive age, affecting between 20% and 50%. While they may cause pressure, abnormal bleeding, and bladder and bowel dysfunction, many cause no symptoms. Fibroids are very rarely the sole cause of infertility.

However, fibroids may impact fertilization by distorting the anatomy of the cervix, altering uterine activity, deforming the uterine cavity, or obstructing the tubal ostia (openings) into the uterine cavity. Implantation may be compromised because of interference with endometrial (uterine lining) development and distortion of the uterine cavity.

It has been reported that only fibroids distorting the uterine cavity significantly impair implantation and pregnancy rates.[1]

Another study observed that fibroids less than seven centimeters in diameter, that did not distort the uterine cavity, did not negatively impact IVF outcomes.[2]

There is mounting evidence indicating that removal of submucosal fibroids improves fertility and reduces recurrent pregnancy loss. The data on the benefits of removing intramural fibroids is less convincing.

Sonohysterogram (transvaginal ultrasound examination with saline contrast) is as sensitive (accurate) as hysteroscopy (looking inside the uterine cavity through the cervical canal via the vagina) in evaluating fibroids that distort the cavity, and it gives a more accurate assessment of their size.

If they are not too large (according to the surgeon's experience), submucosal fibroids warrant serious consideration for removal before IVF treatment.[3] Assessments of outcomes after removal

---

1   Farhi J, Ashkenazi J, Feldberg D, Dicker D, Orvieto R, and Ben Rafael Z. *Effect of uterine leiomyomata on the results of in vitro fertilization treatment.* Hum. Reprod. 1995; 10:2576-2578.
2   Ramzy AM, Sattar M, Amin Y, Mansour RT, Serour GI, and Aboulgar MA. *Uterine fibromyomata and outcome of assisted reproduction.* Hum. Reprod. 1998; 13:198-202.
3   Shokeir T. *Hysteroscopic management in submucous fibroids to improve fertility.* Arch. Gynecol. Obstet. 2005; 273:50-54.

of submucosal fibroids demonstrated not only a dramatic improvement in the live birth rate, but also a very marked reduction in the miscarriage rate.

There are other options for the treatment of intramural fibroids, but their value and benefit await evaluation by randomized prospective trials:

Q Magnetic Resonance Imaging (MRI) guided focused ultrasounds are very expensive, and their value is unproven.

Q Uterine Artery Embolization (UAE) is a radiological procedure that involves injecting very small, inert particles via the uterine artery to block the blood supply to fibroids and make them shrink. It carries a small, but not insignificant, risk of compromising ovarian reserve or inducing premature menopause.

Congenital Uterine Abnormalities

The impact of congenital (present since birth) uterine abnormalities (e.g. a uterine septum) on IVF treatment has only been looked at in a very small number of studies.

One study compared 119 egg collections from 38 women with congenital uterine abnormalities with 7,677 egg collections from the general patient population over the same period of time.[4]

Women who had had a uterine septum (abnormal connective tissue ridge of variable length that divides the uterine cavity) removed had similar pregnancy and implantation rates to

---

4   Lavergne N, Aristizabal J, Zara V, Erny R, and Hebon B. *Uterine abnormalities and in vitro fertilization:what are the results?* Eur.J.Obstet.Gynecol. Reprod. Biol. 1996; 68:29-34.

the general group, while women with untreated septa had 50% lower pregnancy and implantation rates.

Adenomyosis

Adenomyosis is the presence of endometrium (uterine lining) within the myometrium (uterine wall). An MRI study of 152 infertile women revealed that when the innermost part of the uterine wall was abnormally thick, only 2% of embryo transfers resulted in a pregnancy.[5]

A recent meta-analysis showed a reduced clinical pregnancy rate in the presence of adenomyosis in IVF/ICSI treatment cycles.[6]

However, four cases of recurrent implantation failure associated with adenomyosis have been reported that resulted in achieving ongoing pregnancies. They were treated with prolonged down-regulation (turning off the brain's cycling center so that no estrogen is produced by the ovaries) with Zoladex or Synarel (drugs known as GnRH analogues) for six to eight weeks before their next embryo transfer.[7]

5   Maubon A, Faury A, Kapella M, Pouquet M and Piver P. *Uterine junctional zone at magnetic resonance imaging: a predictor of in vitro fertilization implantation failure.* J. Obstet. Gynaecol. Res. 2010; 36:611-618.
6   Vercellini P, Consonni D, Dridi D, Bracco B, Frattaruolo MP, and Somigliana E. *Uterine adenomyosis and in vitro fertilization outcome: a systematic review and meta-analysis.* Hum. Reprod. 2014; 29:964-977.
7   Tremellen K and Russell P. *Adenomyosis is a potential cause of recurrent implantation failure during IVF treatment.* Aust. NZ. J. Obstet. Gynaecol. 2011; 51:280-283.

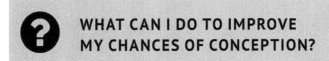

WHAT CAN I DO TO IMPROVE MY CHANCES OF CONCEPTION?

Uterine fibroids are very rarely the only cause of infertility.

Submucosal fibroids can reduce the success of IVF treatment and may contribute to recurrent pregnancy loss. Serious consideration should be given to submucosal fibroid removal before IVF treatment.

Likewise, uterine septa, which are also associated with recurrent pregnancy loss, should be considered for removal before IVF treatment.

Currently, the only treatment that may be helpful when adenomyosis is associated with recurrent implantation failure is an extended course of a GnRH analogue, a medication that will turn off the cycling center in the brain that is responsible for stimulating the ovaries to produce estrogen. Further research is required to confirm the effectiveness of this treatment.

CHAPTER 5

Is It My Lining?

Determination Above All Else

There was no doubt that IVF was the only treatment for Fiona and George, as he had azoospermia (no sperm in his sperm sample) due to a congenital absence of the vas deferens (tubes that transport sperm from the testes to the seminal vesicles, from where they are normally ejaculated via the penis). Their likelihood of successful treatment was high since they were both young; Fiona was 27, and George was 29.

Their first stimulated IVF cycle, involving testicular biopsy under local anesthesia to obtain sperm, was uncomplicated. Only two good quality day five embryos (blastocysts) resulted. One was transferred fresh, and the other was frozen. However, Fiona's period came two days early, and there was no detectable pregnancy hormone when a blood test was performed.

Their fertility specialist recommended a hysteroscopy (looking inside the uterine cavity through the cervical canal via the vagina) before any more embryos were transferred, in order to exclude anything that may have interfered with implantation. The hysteroscopy was performed, but no submucosal fibroids, endometrial polyps, or uterine septa were identified.

An endometrial biopsy (sample of the uterine lining) was taken at the same time. The biopsy revealed chronic endometritis (inflammation of the uterine lining). This was treated with a two-week course of antibiotics. A follow-up endometrial biopsy was performed as an office procedure. The biopsy was normal (i.e. there was no longer evidence of chronic inflammation).

A thawed embryo transfer during the next natural cycle resulted in a pregnancy, but the six week scan revealed a blighted ovum (pregnancy sac within the uterine cavity but no fetus). Three days later, Fiona started bleeding and miscarried.

Fiona and George required counseling, and they took a break before beginning another stimulated cycle.

Another endometrial biopsy was performed to exclude recurrence of the chronic endometritis. It was normal. In their next treatment cycle, Fiona once again stimulated well. George was pleased that there was frozen sperm remaining from the original testicular biopsy. This frozen sperm was thawed and yielded plenty of motile sperm.

Intra-Cytoplasmic Sperm Injection (ICSI) which had also been performed in the first cycle, once again produced a good fertilization rate. However, only one good quality day five embryo (blastocyst) was produced, and it was transferred fresh. Disappointingly, no pregnancy resulted. More supportive counseling was provided.

Their fertility specialist had noted that articles in the medical (infertility) literature were increasingly finding a correlation with premature elevation of serum progesterone (progesterone levels normally rise after ovulation or egg collection) and lower pregnancy rates.

Showing great courage and determination, Fiona and George decided to go ahead with another stimulated cycle following the onset of her next period. Before starting, another endometrial biopsy was performed to exclude recurrent endometritis. It was normal.

Because Fiona's serum progesterone was significantly elevated on the day of hCG trigger injection, a decision was made to freeze all embryos created and to not perform a fresh embryo transfer. Three good quality embryos were frozen on day five.

One embryo was thawed and transferred in Fiona's next natural cycle, again preceded by endometrial biopsy prior to day one of that cycle. Once more, there was no evidence of chronic endometritis.

Finally, a successful pregnancy resulted, and Eliza was born just before Christmas. Fiona and George still have two frozen embryos for future use.

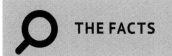

THE FACTS

Endometrial Polyps

The first study on the impact of endometrial polyps (non-cancerous growths within the lining of the uterus) was conducted in 1999, and it concluded that small endometrial polyps (less than two centimeters) do not decrease the pregnancy rate. However, it also discovered a trend towards increased pregnancy loss. According to the authors, "A policy of oocyte retrieval, polypectomy, freezing the embryos, and replacing them in the future might increase the take home baby rate."[1]

Six years later, the first randomized prospective study (where half the patients underwent the procedure and the other half did not) was designed to determine whether polypectomy (removing the polyp) before intrauterine insemination affected pregnancy rates. The pregnancy rate was twice as high in the group that had undergone polypectomy before treatment. The size of the polyp did not have a significant impact on pregnancy rates.[2]

In 2006, two groups of patients were studied; one group had been diagnosed with endometrial polyps during IVF ovulation induction and the other group was made up of patients who had undergone polyp removal before starting their IVF/ICSI cycle or who had no polyps in the first place. This study concluded that "Endometrial polyps discovered during ovulation induction do not negatively affect pregnancy and implantation outcomes in ICSI cycles."[3]

A report in 2012 came to the same conclusion.[4]

There is conflicting evidence about the impact of endometrial polyps on IVF outcomes, but the most recent studies suggest that it is not as important as previously thought.

1   Lass A, Williams G, Abusheikha N, and Brinsden P. *The Effect of Endometrial Polyps on Outcomes of In Vitro Fertilization [IVF] Cycles.* Journal of Assisted Reproduction and Genetics 1999. 16:410-415.
2   Perez-Medina T, Bajo-Arenas J, Salazar F, Redondo T, Sanfrutos L, Alvarez P, and Engels V. *Endometrial polyps and their implication in the pregnancy rates of patients undergoing intrauterine insemination: a prospective randomized study.* Hum. Reprod. 2005; 20:1632-1635.
3   Isikoglou M, Berkkanoglu M, Senturk Z, Coetzee K, and Ozgur K. *Endometrial polyps smaller than 1.5 cm do not affect ICSI outcome.* Reprod. BioMed. Online 2006; 12:199-204.
4   Tiras B, Korucuoglu U, Polat M, Zevneloglu HB, Saltik A, and Yarali H. *Management of endometrial polyps diagnosed before or during ICSI cycles.* Reprod. BioMed. Online 2012; 24:123-128.

Chronic Endometritis

Chronic endometritis is inflammation of the uterine lining, which can be caused by a range of microorganisms. It is usually diagnosed on the basis of the histological finding (looking under a microscope) of plasma cells in the endometrium (uterine lining).

At the Annual Meeting of the American Society for Clinical Pathology in 2005, a paper was presented that demonstrated that a special stain for a substance on the surface of plasma cells was more accurate than the usual methods of identifying them. It reduced the rate of false positive results (due to mistaking mast cells for plasma cells) by 36% and the false negative rate (failing to identify plasma cells) by 40%.[5]

In a study of 106 women with recurrent implantation failure, 45% were confirmed to be suffering from chronic endometritis. After appropriate antibiotic treatment, there was microscopic confirmation of normal endometrium in 75%, while for 25%, chronic endometritis was still present. There were statistically significantly better pregnancy and live birth rates in the former group, whose chronic endometritis had been successfully treated.[6]

A more recent study reported chronic endometritis in 14% of women with recurrent implantation failure and 27% of women with recurrent pregnancy loss.[7]

---

5   Fuentes S. *Immunostain CD 138 May Improve Detection Rate of Chronic Endometritis.* A.S.C.P. Annual Meeting 2005; Abstract 72.
6   Kasius JC, Fatemi HM, Bourgain C, Sie-go DM, Eijkemans RJ, Fauser BC, Devroey P, and Broekmans FJ. *The impact of chronic endometritis on reproductive outcome.* Fertil. Steril. 2011; 96:1451-1456.
7   Cicinelli E, Matteo M, Tinelli R, Lepera A, Alfonso R, Indraccolo U, Marrocchella S, Greco P, and Resta L. *Prevalence of chronic endometritis in repeated unexplained implantation failure and the IVF success rate after antibiotic therapy.* Hum. Reprod. 2015; 30:323-330.

A study in 2014 revealed that women with endometriosis were twice as likely to have chronic endometritis, compared to those who did not have endometriosis.[8]

Tubal Pathology

For more than 20 years, it has been extensively reported that hydrosalpinges (fluid filled blocked fallopian tubes) are associated with low implantation and pregnancy rates in women undergoing IVF treatment. The diseased tubes should be removed or occluded near the uterus because the fluid in diseased tubes may damage embryos if it flows into the uterine cavity.

Intrauterine Fluid

While the accumulation of fluid in the uterine cavity after ovarian stimulation and before embryo transfer is an event that we have long been aware of, it has usually been associated with hydrosalpinges, but this is not always the case.

One study demonstrated that fluid accumulation within the uterine cavity, which had an incidence of 4.7% (35 out of 746), significantly reduced pregnancy rates in women undergoing IVF. Only 2.8% of those with intrauterine fluid became pregnant, compared with 27.1% of women without intrauterine fluid accumulation.[9]

There is no doubt that ovarian stimulation plays an important role in the development and persistence of fluid accumulation because it is not observed in prior unstimulated cycles.

---

8   Takebayashi A, Kimura F, Kishi V, Ishida M, Takahashi A, Yamanaka A, Takahashi K, Suginami H and Murakami T. *The Association between Endometriosis and Chronic Endometritis.* PLOS ONE. February 2014.
9   Chien LW, Au HK, Xiao J, and Tzeng CR. *Fluid accumulation within the uterine cavity reduces pregnancy rates in women undergoing IVF.* Hum. Reprod. 2002; 17:351-356.

Is My Lining Out of Sync?

There is now sufficient evidence to make the determination that elevated serum progesterone on the day of the human Chorionic Hormone (hCG) trigger (to mature eggs prior to collection) in IVF cycles adversely affects outcomes.

Using donor egg cycles, it was proven that a poor outcome is not a result of the effect of elevated progesterone on the egg or embryo.[10]

This finding confirmed that the premature rise in progesterone affects the uterine lining, making it more developmentally mature than the embryo, and, therefore, less receptive to implantation.

This was believed to only be an issue with embryos in the cleavage stage (day two or three) and not with blastocysts (day five embryos). However, a very large study of more than 2,500 patients demonstrated that it is also associated with a lower live birth rate after a day five fresh embryo transfer.[11]

In a meta-analysis of 60,000 stimulated cycles, researchers attempted to determine a threshold (cut off value) for serum progesterone levels, above which outcomes are adversely affected. When all data sets were combined, they found the strongest effect was observed between 1.5 ng/ml and 1.8 ng/ml (4.8 nmol/L and 5.6 nmol/L).[12]

---

10   Melo MA, Mesequer M, Garrido N, Bosch E, Pellicer A, and Remohi J. *The significance of premature luteinisation in an oocyte-donation programme.* Hum. Reprod. 2006; 21: 1503-1507.
11   Ochsenkuhn R, Arzberger A, von Schonfeldt V, Gallwas J, Rogenhofer N, Crispin A, Thaler CJ, and Noss U. *Subtle progesterone rise on the day of hCG administration is associated with lower live birth rates in women undergoing assisted reproductive technology: a retrospective study with 2,555 fresh emryo transfers.* Fertil. Steril. 2012; 98:347-354.
12   Venetis CA, Kolibianakis EM, Bosdou JK, and Tartatzis BC. *Progesterone elevation and probability of pregnancy after IVF: systematic review and meta-analysis of over 60,000 cycles.* Hum. Reprod. Update 2013; 19:433-457.

Endometrial Thickness

A meta-analysis of 22 studies, involving 10,724 cases, addressed the issue of endometrial (uterine lining) thickness and pregnancy rates after IVF.[13]

The incidence of a thin endometrium (equal to or less than seven millimeters) was 2.4%.

A thin endometrium was associated with a clinical pregnancy rate that was less than half of the rate in cases where the endometrium was more than seven millimeters thick.

However, there were variable factors that could not be corrected for that complicated the role of endometrial thickness in implantation.

The authors felt that, based on the available evidence, endometrial thickness alone should not be used to decide whether to proceed with embryo transfer or not.

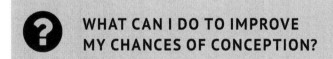

WHAT CAN I DO TO IMPROVE MY CHANCES OF CONCEPTION?

The jury is still out on the role of endometrial polyps as it relates to IVF treatment outcomes.

It is important to exclude chronic endometritis because it compromises the prospects of a good outcome.

13   Kasius A, Smit JG, Torrance HL, Eijkemans MJ, Mol BW, Opmeer BC, Broekmans FJ. *Endometrial thickness and pregnancy rates after IVF:a systematic review and Meta-analysis.* Hum. Reprod. Update 2014; 20:530-541.

The presence of blocked, fluid-filled fallopian tubes significantly reduces the success of IVF treatment. There is no doubt that they should be removed or occluded near the uterus before any IVF treatment.

If serum progesterone is elevated on the day of the hCG trigger, a fresh embryo transfer would seem unwise and all embryos should be frozen for transfer in a subsequent natural or artificial (medically induced with estrogen and progesterone in the form of pills, pessaries, patches or injections) cycle.

CHAPTER 6

Is It My Endometriosis?

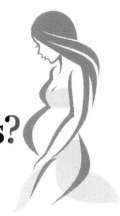

Preserving Ovarian Reserve

It had been eight years since Michelle's first laparoscopy for typical symptoms of endometriosis. Since then, she had undergone five more. The most recent had been nine months prior, three months after she met Michael, because of pain during intercourse.

They were now in a serious relationship, and a family was on their immediate life agenda.

Michael had a sperm test, which proved to be normal. Michelle's hormone tests indicated that she was ovulating. Her last laparoscopy had shown that her tubes were open and healthy. Michelle was 30 years of age, and Michael was 32.

They were referred to a fertility specialist because they wanted to work out a plan. They were worried that Michelle's past history of endometriosis and multiple surgeries for the condition might make it more difficult for them for conceive.

Michelle's ovarian reserve (her ovaries' ability to produce fertilizable eggs) became the focus of attention. Her Anti-Mullerian

Hormone (AMH) was 1.4 nmol/ml (10 pmol/L), and her Antral Follicle Count (AFC) was 8. These results were at the lower limit of normal. It was suggested that they try on their own for 6 months and, if unsuccessful, proceed to IVF.

Time passed, but no pregnancy.

Before starting their first stimulated IVF cycle, Michelle had an ultrasound examination that revealed bilateral two-centimeter ovarian endometriomas (benign cysts lined by the same cells as her uterine cavity). This indicated that there was a high likelihood that multiple small areas of the pelvis were affected by endometriosis.

Their fertility specialist advised against surgery because Michelle currently had no pain and there was a risk of more ovarian surgery further compromising her ovarian reserve.

He did, however, recommend a three-month course of a Gonadotrophin Releasing Hormone (GnRH) agonist prior to beginning on IVF treatment. This would stop Michelle's brain from releasing hormones stimulating her ovaries to produce estrogen, which promotes and maintains the growth of endometriosis. The endometriotic deposits would consequently shrink. It was explained that this treatment was unlikely to have any significant effect on the endometriomas but that it was believed to improve IVF treatment results.

Three months after having her GnRH agonist hormone implant, Michelle commenced a long down-regulated treatment cycle. This entailed continuing to use a GnRH agonist (as a nasal spray) and starting Follicle Stimulating Hormone (FSH) injections to make the follicles grow and eggs develop before hCG triggering to ripen her eggs prior to collection.

Eight mature egg were retrieved, six fertilized normally, and two good quality day five embryos (blastocysts) were produced. One was transferred fresh, and the other was frozen.

A normal ongoing pregnancy resulted.

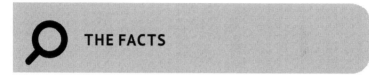

THE FACTS

A study published in 2005 revealed that severe endometriosis meant a worse prognosis for IVF/ICSI treatments, compared to milder disease or tubal factors.[1]

Subsequently, a systematic review and meta-analysis investigating the effect of surgical treatment for endometriomas (ovarian cysts lined with the same cells as the uterine cavity) on IVF outcomes found there was no significant difference between the treated and untreated groups.[2]

A report on IVF outcomes in women with unoperated bilateral endometriomas found that the quality of eggs collected and the chances of pregnancy were not affected.[3]

In 2015, a systematic review of 1,346 articles published between 1980 and 2014 resulted in a meta-analysis that concluded,

1   Kulvasaari P, Hippelainen M, and Heinonen S. *Effect of endometriosis on IVF/ICSI outcome: stage 111/1V endometriosis worsens cumulative pregnancy and live-born rates.* Hum. Reprod. 2005; 20:3130-3135.
2   Tsoumpou I, Kyrgiou M, Gelbaya TA, and Nardo LG. *The effect of surgical treatment for endometrioma on in vitro fertilization outcomes: a systematic review and meta-analysis.* Fertil, Steril. 2009;92:75-87.
3   Benaglia L, Bermejo A, Somigliani E, Faulisi S, Ragni G, Fedele L, and Garcia-Velasco JA. *In vitro fertilization outcome in women with unoperated bilateral endometriomas.* Fertil. Steril. 2013; 99:1714-1719.

"Women with and without endometriosis have comparable outcomes in terms of live births, whereas those with severe endometriosis have inferior outcomes. There is insufficient evidence to recommend surgery routinely before undergoing ART." [4]

The most recent systematic review and meta-analysis (2016) not only agreed with the conclusions of the 2015 review, but also added, "Even after surgical removal of endometriosis, IVF-ET (embryo transfer) results remain worse than controls."[5]

A Cochrane Collaboration Systematic Review also came to the same conclusion. Surgical removal of endometriomas prior to IVF was not supported, and a poorer response to controlled ovarian hyperstimulation was noted in the group that underwent surgery.[6]

However, the same Cochrane Collaboration Systematic Review did conclude that "based on currently available evidence, women with endometriosis treated with IVF or ICSI should receive GnRH agonist therapy for a minimum of three months prior to the procedure as this will increase the odds of clinical pregnancy fourfold."

Sepsis after egg collection is rare. It almost always occurs when ovarian endometriomas are accidentally punctured and

---

4   Hamdan M, Omar S, Dunselman G, and Cheong Y. *Influece of Endometriosis on Assisted Reproductive Technology Outcomes: A Systematic Review and Meta-Analysis.* Obstet. Gynecol. 2015; 125:79-88.
5   Rossi AC and Prefumo F. *The effect of surgery for endometriosis on pregnancy outcomes following in vitro fertilization: a systematic review and meta-analysis.* Arch. Gynecol. Obstet. 2016; 294:647-655.
6   Sallam HN, Garcia Velasco JA, Dias S, Arici A, and Abou-Setta AM. *Long-term pituitary down-regulation before in vitro fertilization(IVF) for women with endometriosis.* Cochrane Collaboration Systematic Review. 2010.

vaginal bacteria introduced into the cyst by the egg collection needle passing through the vaginal wall.[7]

This risk can be minimized by giving preventative (prophylactic) antibiotics at the time of egg collection.

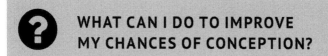

❓ WHAT CAN I DO TO IMPROVE MY CHANCES OF CONCEPTION?

Minimal or mild endometriosis is unlikely to adversely affect your IVF treatment outcome, but severe (especially infiltrating) endometriosis will.

There is a strong case for not operating on endometriomas because surgical intervention is likely to reduce the ovarian reserve, the response to ovarian stimulation, and therefore, the number of eggs collected. There is also no good evidence that such surgery will improve outcomes. If you have ovarian endometriomas, it would be best to leave them alone, unless they are causing you significant symptoms.

If you have endometriosis, an extended course of a GnRH agonist prior to starting an IVF stimulated cycle will have a positive impact on the outcome.

7   Benaglia L, Somigliana E, Iemmello R, Colpi E, Nicolosi AE, and Ragni G. *Endometrioma and oocyte retrieval induced pelvic abscess: a clinical concern or an exceptional complication.* Fertil. Steril. 2008; 89:1263-1266.

CHAPTER 7

Is It My Immune System?

A Difficult Choice

Christine was 40 years of age, and her partner, Tom, was 32. They very much wanted to have a baby together. After trying to conceive naturally for five months without success, they decided to proceed directly to IVF.

Tom's sperm test was normal. Christine's ovarian reserve (capacity of her ovaries to produce fertilizable eggs) was surprisingly good, meaning she should respond well to ovarian stimulation in an IVF treatment cycle.

After three stimulated cycles with fresh embryo transfers and five natural cycles with thawed embryo transfers, a total of 11 cleavage stage (day two or three) embryos had been transferred, but there was still no ongoing pregnancy. The couple had been advised that embryos were better off in utero at day two or three, than in culture medium until day five.

Their fertility specialist suggested autoimmune screening for Christine. It revealed a positive result for Anti-Phospholipid Antibodies (APA) and an abnormally high number of uterine Natural Killer (uNK) cells.

Heparin injections (a blood thinner that can have a suppressive effect on the immune system) and prednisolone tablets (a corticosteroid, a type of drug that suppresses the immune system) were included in the next stimulated cycle.

Two day two embryos were created and transferred fresh. Unfortunately, no pregnancy resulted. Christine and Tom requested a second opinion.

It was suggested that Pre-implantation Genetic Screening (PGS) be performed in their next stimulated cycle. This would ensure that they avoid transferring aneuploid (chromosomally abnormal) embryos, which are very unlikely to result in an ongoing pregnancy.

They returned to their original fertility specialist for further treatment. Christine once again stimulated well. Seven embryos resulted that were suitable for biopsy on day three but by day five, only one had survived. However, the chromosomal analyses of all seven embryos were very abnormal, so the lone surviving day five embryo was not transferred.

It became apparent to Christine and Tom that the most likely explanation for their lack of success with IVF thus far was the high proportion of chromosomally abnormal eggs that Christine was producing due to her age.

After several counseling sessions, they came to terms with the fact that the use of donor oocytes or donor embryos offered them the best prospect of achieving their dream (see Chapter 15).

Their first recipient IVF treatment cycle used a 32-year-old egg donor. Only a single embryo was transferred because of the donor's age, as there was a significant risk of multiple pregnancy if more than one embryo was transferred. The transfer resulted in an ongoing singleton pregnancy.

An ultrasound examination and blood tests didn't reveal any suggestion of fetal chromosomal abnormalities, and the 18 week scan showed no major anatomical abnormalities.

James was born at 38 weeks.

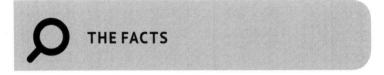

THE FACTS

Anti-Phospholipid Antibody (APA)

In 2000, a meta-analysis evaluated the effect of Anti-Phospholipid Antibodies (APA) on the likelihood of IVF success and concluded that testing for APA was not justified for patients undergoing IVF.[1]

The Practice Committee of the American Society for Reproductive Medicine (ASRM) stated in 2008 that there is no association between APA abnormalities and IVF success; therefore, there is no justification for assessment or treatment of APA in couples undergoing IVF, on the basis of currently available information. There has been no reason for ASRM to change its viewpoint because, in the last nine years, there has been no new evidence to support this type of testing.

---

1   Hornstein MD, Davis OK, Massey JB, Paulson RJ, and Collins JA. *Antiphospholipid antibodies and in vitro fertilization success: a meta-analysis.* Fertil. Steril. 2000; 73:330-333.

Uterine Natural Killer (uNK) Cells

It should be highlighted that uterine Natural Killer (uNK) cells were only one in a range of immune and vascular abnormalities found in the endometria (uterine lining) of women with recurrent implantation failure.[2]

A recent systematic review of the literature stated, "This review does not support the use of prednisolone, IVg (intravenous gamma-globulin), or any other adjuvant treatment in women undergoing ART (Assisted Reproductive Technology) who are found to have elevated absolute numbers or activity of uNK cells, purely due to the absence of, or poor quality, of the evidence."[3]

In 2014, another meta-analysis of studies evaluating the role of uNK cells in regards to IVF outcome concluded by stating: "On the basis of current evidence, uNK cell analysis and immune therapy should be offered only in the context of clinical research."[4]

Another excellent review of studies involving corticosteroid therapy in assisted reproduction, published in 2016, argued, "unless overt immune pathology is evident, utilization of corticosteroids is not warranted and may be harmful."[5]

2   Quenby S and Farquharson R. *Uterine natural killer cells, implantation failure and recurrent miscarriage.* Reprod. BioMed. Online 2006; 13:24-28.
3   Polanski LT, Barbosa MAP, Martins WP, Baumgarten MN, Campbell B, Brosens J, Quenby S, and Raine-Fleming N. *Interventions to improve reproductive outcomes in women with elevated natural killer cells undergoing assisted reproduction techniques: a systematic review of literature.* Hum. Reprod. 2014;29:65-75.
4   Sashadri S and Sunkara SK. *Natural killer cells in female infertility and recurrent miscarriage: a systematic review and meta-analysis.* Hum Reprod. Update 2014; 20:429-438.
5   Robertson SA, Jin M, Yu D, Moldenhauer LM, Davis MJ, and Norman RJ. *Corticosteroid therapy in assisted reproduction-immune suppression is a faulty premise.* Hum. Reprod. 2016; 31:2164-2173.

The most recent review, in 2017, concluded that, "The current evidence base does not support the clinical use of immunomodulation therapies in patients undergoing IVF."[6]

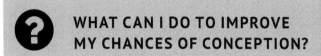

WHAT CAN I DO TO IMPROVE MY CHANCES OF CONCEPTION?

Conducting blood tests for autoimmune diseases, including antiphospholipid antibodies, does not seem to be useful. Additionally, treatment when positive results are found is not justified in the case of IVF treatment, based on available evidence.

There is currently no reason to test for uterine Natural Killer cells because it remains to be established what actually constitutes an abnormal number of these cells and how they might affect conception. There is currently no scientific basis for treatment.

Do not subject yourself to the possible side effects of medication that has no proven value.

---

6   Hvlid MM and Macklon N. *Immune modulation treatments = where is the evidence?* Fertil. Steril. 2017; 107:1284-1293.

CHAPTER 8

Is It His Sperm?

So Who Is The Problem?

Harry was 35 and overweight. He smoked and met his friends for a few drinks after work every day. He also did not exercise. He loved his partner, Sally, a 32 year-old non-smoker who had only a very occasional glass of wine. Sally also exercised sensibly and maintained a healthy weight. She encouraged Harry to change his lifestyle, but so far, she had been unsuccessful.

Pregnancy eluded them, even though Sally had a regular menstrual cycle and they made love several times a week.

They saw their family physician (general practitioner), who arranged for Sally to have a blood test to confirm she was ovulating and an ultrasound examination to make sure that her fallopian tubes were open and that there were no other abnormalities that might interfere with her getting pregnant. A sperm test was organized for Harry.

Sally was ovulating and her tubes were open, but Harry's sperm test was far from normal. The sperm test was repeated, and the second result was even worse.

They were told that their best chance of achieving a pregnancy was IVF with ICSI, Intra-Cytoplasmic Sperm Injection (injecting individual sperm into individual eggs).

The Next Step

Sally and Harry were referred to a fertility specialist, who agreed that IVF with ICSI may be necessary but insisted that Harry make lifestyle changes before proceeding down this path. Sally was thrilled that the fertility specialist shared her sentiments. Harry agreed, somewhat reluctantly, to change his ways.

Four months of weight reduction (through diet and exercise), abstinence from alcohol, and quitting smoking had its ups and downs for the couple, but their relationship survived.

A follow up sperm test was normal!

Sally conceived naturally the next month.

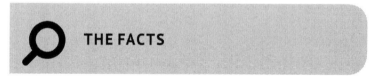

THE FACTS

Obesity

Obesity is a high oxidative (cell damaging) stress.[1] Oxidative stress is the leading cause of DNA fragmentation (damage to genetic material) in sperm.[2] The greater the level of DNA fragmentation in sperm, the worse the outcome of IVF treatment.[3]

1   Luke B, Brown MB, Missmer SA, Bukulmez O, Leach R, and Stern JE. *The effect of obesity on response to and outcome of assisted reproductive technology: a national survey;* Fertil. Steril. 2011; 96:820-825.
2   Aitken RJ, De Julius GN, Finnie JM, Hedges A, and McLachlan RL. *Analysis of the relationship between oxidative stress, DNA damage and sperm vitality in a patient population development of diagnostic criteria.* Hum. Reprod. 2010; 25:2415-2426.
3   Zhang Y, Wang H, Wang I, Zhou Z, Sha J, Mao Y, Cai L, Feng T, Yan Z, Ma L, and Liu J. *The clinical significance of sperm DNA damage detection combined with routine semen testing in assisted reproduction.* Mol. Med. Rep. 2008; 1:617-624.

Both moderate exercise and weight reduction have been shown to improve sperm test results.[4]

Smoking

If the male partner smokes, it has a significant negative effect on IVF/ICSI outcome, reducing the live birth rate from 21.1% to 7.8%.[5]

If the male partner smokes and the female partner is exposed to the second-hand smoke, the pregnancy rate is impacted drastically—20.0%, compared to 48.3% in women who are not exposed to cigarette smoke.[6]

Alcohol

Men who consume beer daily were 27% more likely to have poor quality sperm.

Weekly white wine consumption was associated with a 43% increase in the likelihood of poor sperm morphology (shape), and red wine increased the odds of a low sperm count by 23%.[7]

Azoospermia (no sperm)

The total absence of sperm in the ejaculate may be due to obstruction, for example, past history of vasectomy or congenital absence of vas deferens (absence of the tubes that take sperm from the testicles to the seminal vesicles from

---

4   Sharma R, Biedenharm KR, Fedor JM, and Agarwal A. *Lifestyle factors and reproductive health: taking control of your fertility.* Reprod. Biol. Endocrinol. 2011; 11:66.
5   Fuentes A, Munoz A, Barnhart K, Arguello B, Diaz M, and Pommer R. *Recent smoking and reproductive technologies outcome.* Fertil. Steril. 2010; 93[1]:89-89.
6   Neal MS, Hughes EG, Holloway AC, and Foster WG. *Sidestream smoking is equally as damaging as mainstream smoking on IVF outcomes.* Hum. Reprod. 2005; 20[9]:2531-2531.
7   Rossi BV, Berry KF, Hornstein MD, Cramer DW, Ehrlich S, and Missmer S. *Effect of alcohol on in vitro fertilization.* Obstet. Gynecol. 2011; 117[1]:136-142.

which they are ejaculated via the penis). This can be treated by IVF with ICSI, using sperm obtained by testicular needle biopsy under local anesthetic. If it is due to testicular failure, donor sperm is the only treatment option.

Rarely, it is due to a chromosomal abnormality. (One such example is Klinefelter's Syndrome, which results when a man has an extra X chromosome. This gives him an XXY chromosomal pattern, compared with a typical XY male). This condition is associated with very small testes. Under these circumstances, it is sometimes possible to obtain a very small number of sperm suitable for IVF/ICSI through open microsurgical testicular biopsy under general anesthesia. Normal pregnancies have resulted.

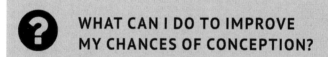

❓ WHAT CAN I DO TO IMPROVE MY CHANCES OF CONCEPTION?

The male partner's lifestyle can significantly impact sperm quality and negatively influence the outcome of IVF treatment.

Encourage your partner to lead a healthy lifestyle.

CHAPTER 9

Was It My Embryo Transfer?

Past History Matters

Kathy, 31, and her partner, Paul, 33, decided to try IVF because, after 9 months of trying to conceive, their failure to conceive remained unresolved and unexplained, despite thorough investigation.

Six years prior, Kathy had undergone laser treatment for high-grade pre-cancerous changes to her cervix. No recurrent abnormality had been detected during her regular six-monthly follow up appointments, which involved repeat smear tests and colposcopies (looking at the cervix with a magnifying instrument). She had gone back to having a smear test once every two years.

First IVF Cycle

In their first stimulated IVF treatment cycle, the creation of four good quality day five embryos (blastocysts) was considered to be a very good outcome. Fresh embryo transfer, however, proved to be technically difficult.

Cervical stenosis (narrowing of the cervical canal) due to scar tissue from her laser treatment made it impossible to pass the outer embryo transfer catheter and required cervical dilatation (opening up the cervical canal with an instrument).

There was also uterine retroversion (the body of uterus was lying behind, rather than in front of, the cervix). This made it necessary to grasp the cervix with a tenaculum (long metal pincer forceps) and pull it down the vagina so that the body of the uterus became horizontally aligned with the cervix (i.e. the cervical canal was in the same plane as the uterine cavity).

A small amount of active bleeding from the cervical canal was observed. Eventually, the outer catheter was inserted just inside the uterine cavity, enabling placement of the inner catheter carrying the embryo into the uterine cavity. The embryo was then injected into the cavity. Upon removal, both the inside and outside of the inner catheter were slightly bloody.

Ten days later, the pregnancy blood test was negative.

The Next Step

Cervical dilatation (stretching the cervical opening and canal) to make introduction of the embryo transfer catheter easier was performed in conjunction with a trial embryo transfer (a practice embryo transfer procedure without using an embryo) under ultrasound control in the week prior to day one of the natural cycle in which one of the frozen embryos was to be thawed and transferred.

The thawed embryo transfer was performed easily, without any instrumentation, under ultrasound control five days after ovulation.

This time, ten days after the embryo transfer, the pregnancy hormone levels looked very promising. The six week scan revealed a normal ongoing pregnancy.

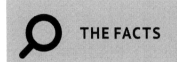

THE FACTS

A very recent study analyzing 7,714 embryo transfers found that a difficult transfer reduces the clinical pregnancy rate by 11% and the live birth rate by 9%.[1]

Holding the cervix with a tenaculum should be avoided, if at all possible, because stimulating the cervix in this manner causes release of a hormone (oxytocin) that increases uterine contractions.[2] This could result in expulsion of the transferred embryo from the uterine cavity.

Embryo transfer catheter placement has a major impact on implantation and pregnancy rates, with catheter placement in the upper or middle uterine cavity, more than one centimeter from the fundus, resulting in the best outcomes.[3]

Immediate embryo transfer catheter withdrawal after embryo expulsion into the uterine cavity does not compromise IVF treatment outcomes.[4]

1   Kava-Braverman A, Martinez F, Rodriguez I, Alvarez M, Barri PN, and Coroleu B. *What is a difficult transfer? Analysis of 7,714 embryo trnasfers: the impact of maneuvers during embryo transfers on pregnancy rate and a proposal of objective assessment.* Fertil. Steril. 2017;107:657-663.

2   Dorn C, Reinsberg J, Schlebusch, Prietl G, Van der Ven H, and Krebs D. *Serum oxytocin concentration during embryo transfer procedure.* Eur. J. Obstet. Gynecol. Reprod. Biol. 1999; 87:77-80.

3   Kwon H, Choi DH, and Kim EK. *Absolute position versus relative position in embryo transfer: a randomized controlled trial.* Reprod. Biol. Endocrinol 2015; 13:78-

4   Sroga JM, Montville CP, Aubuchon M, Williams DB, and Thomas MA. *Effect of delayed versus immediate embryo transfer catheter removal on pregnancy outcomes during fresh cycles.* Fertil. Steril. 2010; 93:2088-2090.

Removing mucus from the endocervical canal seems to improve pregnancy and live birth rates.[5]

Recent meta-analyses (2015 and 2016) provide good evidence that ultrasound-guided embryo transfers improve clinical pregnancy and live birth rates.[6, 7]

In contrast to true active bleeding during or after embryo transfer, the presence of blood on the embryo transfer catheter after its withdrawal does not appear to impact implantation or pregnancy rates.[8, 9]

If an embryo is retained in the embryo transfer catheter (in other words, not expelled) but immediately retransferred, clinical pregnancy rates are not compromised.[10]

There is no evidence to recommend bed rest after embryo transfer.[11]

5   Moini A, Kiani K, Bahmanabadi A, Akhoond M, and Akhlagi A. *Improvement in pregnancy rate by removal of cervical discharge prior to embryo transfer in ICSI cycles: a randomised clinical trial.* Aust. NZ. J Obstet. Gynaecol. 2011; 51:315-32.
6   Texeira DM, Dassuncao LA, Vieira CV, Barbosa MA, Coelho Neto MA, Nastri Co and Martins WP. *Ultrasound guidance during embryo transfer: a systematic review and meta-analysis of randomised controlled trials.* Ultrasound Obstet. Gynecol. 2015; 45:139-148.
7   Brown J, Buckingham K, Buckett W, and Abou-Setta AM. *Ultrasound versus 'clinical touch' for catheter guidance during embryo transfer in women.* Cochrane Collaboration Systematic Review. 2016.
8   Listijono DR, Boylan T, Cooke S, Kilani S, and Chapman MG. *An analysis of the impact of embryo transfer difficulty on live births, using a standardised grading system.* Hum. Fertil. 2013; 16:211-214.
9   Phillips JA, Martins WP, Nastri CO, and Raine-Fenning NJ. *Difficult embryo transfers or blood on catheter and assisted reproductive outcomes: systematic review and meta-analysis.* Eur .J. Obstet. Gynecol. Reprod Biol. 2013; 168:121-128.
10   Yi HJ, Koo HS, Cha SH, Kim HO, Park CW, and Song IO. *Reproductive outcomes of retransferring retained embryos in blastocyst transfer cycles.* Clin. Exp. Reprod. Med. 2016; 43:133-138.
11   Craciunas L and Tsampras N. *Bed rest following embryo transfer might negatively affect the outcome of IVF/ICSI: a systematic review and meta-analysis.* Hum. Fertil. 2016; 19:16-22.

❓ WHAT CAN I DO TO IMPROVE MY CHANCES OF CONCEPTION?

All possible steps must be taken to minimize difficulties at the time of the embryo transfer.

A trial embryo transfer, ideally under ultrasound control, should identify any potential problems.

It can be beneficial to remove cervical mucus from the cervical canal, but care is required to avoid causing bleeding.

Embryo transfers should be performed under ultrasound control.

There is no evidence to recommend bed rest after an embryo transfer.

An embryo transfer, without instrumentation or manipulation, performed under ultrasound control is best practice for successful IVF treatment.

CHAPTER 10

Is It My Stimulation Protocol?

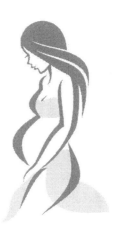

First Cycle

A couple in their early 30s, Ella and Gary, embarked on their first IVF treatment cycle after their unexplained primary infertility had not been resolved by two cycles of ovulation induction and intrauterine insemination.

Their first cycle was a Gonadotrophin Releasing Hormone (GnRH) antagonist cycle.

Daily Follicle Stimulating Hormone (FSH) injections were used to recruit and grow follicles. GnRH antagonist injections were started once the follicles were actively growing. A single injection of Ovidrel, recombinant human Chorionic Gonadotrophin (hCG), 6500 I.U., was the trigger used to mature (ripen) the eggs before collection.

Twelve eggs were collected (four mature and eight immature), despite the fact that 15 follicles were good-sized and should have contained more mature eggs. Two of the mature eggs fertilized normally, but neither embryo grew to day five (blastocyst).

Second Cycle

A different stimulation protocol (known as flare or boost) was utilized. The same dose of FSH was used, but a GnRH agonist (GnRHa) was included from the beginning of the cycle. The latter recruits follicles by stimulating the release of FSH from the pituitary gland.

Once the natural store of FSH is depleted, the agonist stops eggs from being released before egg collection by suppressing the release of Luteinizing Hormone (LH) from the pituitary gland, which would cause ovulation.

Ovidrel was once again employed as the trigger.

Twelve eggs were collected, six of which were mature. Intra-Cytoplasmic Sperm Injection (ICSI) was employed in an attempt to maximize the fertilization rate.

Three embryos were created. Only one of these embryos grew to day five and was transferred fresh, but a pregnancy did not result.

Third Cycle

Ella and Gary's fertility specialist suggested seeking a second opinion, getting counseling, and taking a three-month break from treatment.

The second opinion recommended a long down-regulated cycle, which involved taking the oral contraceptive pill, starting during the period preceding the stimulated cycle. The GnRH agonist (GnRHa) spray was to be commenced during the last week on the pill (incidentally providing control over when the stimulated cycle could be started) and continued until the day of the trigger injection. A higher dose of hCG trigger and a higher dose of FSH for stimulation were also recommended.

Ella and Gary had developed a very good rapport with their original fertility specialist and were impressed with her willingness to have another fertility specialist look at their case from a fresh point of view, so they returned to her for further treatment.

Using the suggested stimulation protocol and trigger, 14 eggs were collected, ten of which were mature. Seven fertilized normally with ICSI. Two good quality day five embryos (blastocysts) resulted. One was transferred fresh on day five, and the other was frozen.

An ongoing pregnancy resulted from the transfer.

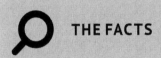

THE FACTS

Currently, the most popular stimulation protocol is a GnRH antagonist cycle with FSH stimulation and an hCG trigger. In this type of cycle, if there is a significant risk of severe Ovarian Hyperstimulation Syndrome (OHSS), hCG can be replaced with a GnRH agonist trigger.

Use of the latter precludes a fresh embryo transfer because the luteal phase (post egg collection) endometrium (uterine lining) that develops is unfavourable for embryo implantation, but the risk of severe OHSS is eliminated.

If the risk of severe OHSS is a concern, fresh embryo transfer should not be considered, and all embryos should be frozen because pregnancy would result in hCG production, with the risk of development of late onset OHSS.

The antagonist cycle is a short, user-friendly, stimulation that, according to the Cochrane Collaboration Systematic Review, has comparable pregnancy, implantation, and live birth rates to long down-regulated stimulation.[1]

However, results are not as good if preceded by use of the oral contraceptive pill to schedule the stimulated cycle.[2]

Prior to the availability of GnRH antagonists, the worldwide stimulation of choice was a long down-regulated cycle, starting with a GnRH agonist seven days before day one of the stimulated cycle and continuing until the hCG trigger. It was sometimes associated with the formation of ovarian cysts, which led to cycle cancellation.

This could be avoided by incorporating the oral contraceptive pill before the stimulated cycle (i.e. as part of the down-regulation phase). However, this type of cycle carries a risk of OHSS in at-risk patients because there is no alternative to the hCG trigger.

This still remains the stimulation protocol of choice when scheduling with the oral contraceptive is necessary for IVF clinics, which only perform certain procedures (e.g. embryo biopsy) on specific days or for optimal clinical efficiency when egg collection is restricted to certain days.

1   Al-Inany HG, Youssef MA, Ayeleke R, Brown J, Lam W and Broekmans FJ. *Gonadotrophin-releasing hormone antagonists versus GnRH agonist in subfertile couples undergoing assisted reproductive technology.* Cochrane Collaboration Systematic Review. 2016.
2   Griesinger G, Kolibianakis EM, Venetis V, Diedrich K, and Tarlatzis B. *Oral contraceptive pretreatment significantly reduces ongoing pregnancy likelihood in gonadotrophin-releasing hormone antagonist cycles: an updated meta-analysis.* Fertil. Steril. 2010; 94:2382-2384.

Before research demonstrated that long down-regulation generally had better outcomes, the flare (or boost) stimulation protocol was favored, based on the belief that the initial release of gonadotrophin (FSH) from the pituitary gland in response to using GnRHa early in the cycle resulted in follicle recruitment.

Daily FSH injections would then recruit even more follicles and promote their growth. In the meantime, continued daily administration of GnRHa would prevent premature release of eggs before the hCG trigger. But, once again, there was concern about OHSS for at-risk patients. Scheduling with the oral contraceptive pill may have also negatively impacted the outcome.

A reanalysis of the Cochrane Database Systematic Review was performed. It excluded both low-dose FSH long, down-regulated protocols and reports from clinics with poor pregnancy rates, suggesting either poor-quality treatment or inclusion of patients with a poor prognosis.

This approach was rationalized on the grounds that simply being a Randomized Controlled Study (RCT) is not enough to justify the inclusion of a poor quality study in a meta-analysis. The reanalysis concluded that long down-regulation resulted in better outcomes.[3]

While hCG 10,000 I.U. is the most commonly used trigger in the USA, Ovidrel (recombinant hCG) equivalent to 6,500 I.U. hCG is the usual trigger in Australia. The former has a higher chance of aggravating OHSS in at-risk patients, but it may be more effective when it comes to final egg maturation, resulting in fewer immature eggs (which will not fertilize) being collected.

---

3   Orvieto R and Patrizio P. *GnRH agonist versus GnRH antagonist in ovarian stimulation: an ongoing debate.* Reprod. BioMed. Online 2013; 26:4-8.

Eggs can be collected during a three-hour window, 35 to 38 hours after the hCG trigger, without compromising results. Therefore, you should not be unduly concerned if the clinic's egg collection schedule is running a little late.[4]

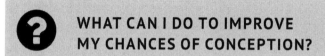

WHAT CAN I DO TO IMPROVE MY CHANCES OF CONCEPTION?

There is no one-size-fits-all ovarian stimulation protocol.

While a GnRH antagonist cycle is user-friendly and appears to have comparable live birth rates to down-regulated cycles, other protocols should be considered if the outcomes have been suboptimal.

4   Weiss A, Neril R, Geslevich J, Lavee M, Beck-Fruchter R, Golan J, and Shalev E. *Lag time from ovulation trigger to oocyte aspiration and oocyte maturity in assisted reproductive technology cycles: a retrospective study.* Fertil. Steril. 2014; 102:419-423.

CHAPTER 11

Why Was There Total Fertilization Failure?

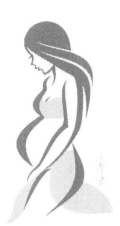

Unexplained Infertility

Peta and Sean, who were both 35, had been trying to have a baby for eight months without any luck. In fact, they wanted to have at least two children.

Extensive investigation resulted in a diagnosis of unexplained infertility.

They decided against ovulation induction and intrauterine insemination as their initial treatment and opted to proceed directly to IVF.

First IVF Cycle

In their first stimulated IVF cycle, ten mature eggs were collected, but none fertilized.

Second IVF Cycle

Eight of the eggs collected in their second cycle were mature. Intra-Cytoplasmic Sperm Injection (ICSI) was employed to avoid another cycle of Total Failed Fertilization (TFF). However, once again, none of the eggs fertilized.

Peta and Sean did not wish to use donor eggs, sperm, or embryos to achieve a pregnancy, but they were willing to try a third and final treatment cycle before abandoning IVF.

Third Cycle

Artificial Oocyte Activation (a technique used to stimulate activity within the egg to encourage fertilization) was incorporated in their final ICSI treatment cycle. A total of nine mature eggs was retrieved; six of these fertilized normally, and two good-quality day five embryos (blastocysts) resulted. One blastocyst was transferred fresh, and the other was frozen.

A normal ongoing pregnancy was finally achieved.

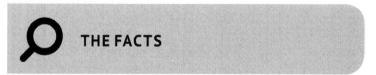

THE FACTS

Total Fertilization Failure (TFF) is a devastating outcome and a very complex issue. It requires discussion with your fertility specialist.

There will be no mature eggs to fertilize if there is a block in egg development between the Germinal Vesicle phase (very early development) and Metaphase 1 (the next stage of development), or at any point between Metaphase 1 and Metaphase 11 (the final stage of development).

Total Fertilization Failure occurs in 5 to 10% of IVF cycles and 1 to 3% of ICSI cycles.

ICSI can overcome problems with sperm-egg interaction (sperm attaching to and/or penetrating the shell of the egg), sperm-egg fusion (sperm getting inside the egg to combine its genetic material with that of the egg), and polyspermy (multiple sperm getting into one egg), when TFF occurs during IVF.

However, when ICSI fails, there may be another problem with the sperm, the eggs, or both. The main cause of ICSI TFF is failure of egg activation. This activation would normally allow the M11 arrested (waiting to develop) egg to continue its development. Egg activation is a complex process and may not be able to take place until the cytoplasm (the part of the egg outside the nucleus, the latter containing the genetic material) is fully developed.

While there are ways of establishing whether activation failure is due to a sperm or egg abnormality, discussion of these methods is beyond the scope of this book. These and other TFF issues are discussed in detail by Catherine Combelles in her review of the subject, which includes 98 references.[1]

Artificial Oocyte Activation can be performed using a modified ICSI technique or calcium ionospheres (special molecules that stir up activity).

Since only mature eggs can be fertilized, a failure of eggs to mature to M11 will prevent fertilization; currently, the only treatment for this problem is the use of donor eggs.

---

1 Combelles C. *Unique Patient Issues; Early Interventions and Management.* Semin. Reprod. Med. 2012; 30:243-252.

Similarly, the use of donor sperm is currently the only solution if the cause of TFF is a structural defect affecting all of the sperm.

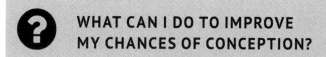

WHAT CAN I DO TO IMPROVE MY CHANCES OF CONCEPTION?

Total fertilization failure is one of the most devastating events in IVF treatment, but it may be possible to treat it without using donor eggs, sperm, or embryos.

TFF requires consultation with your fertility specialist, often in conjunction with an embryologist from the laboratory where the event occurred.

You need to fully understand why TFF has occurred and what your options are in dealing with this enormous disappointment.

CHAPTER 12

Was It My Luteal Phase Support?

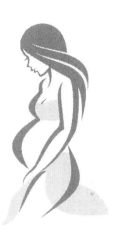

There is no case study to introduce this chapter because it is very rare that inadequate luteal phase support is the primary cause of IVF treatment failure.

However, the medication used, route of administration, and duration of treatment do warrant discussion, as does the addition of a Gonadotrophin Releasing Hormone (GnRH) agonist to fresh embryo transfer cycles to optimize treatment outcomes.

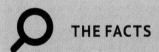 **THE FACTS**

There is no dispute that Luteal Phase Support (LPS) is essential during stimulated IVF treatment cycles that incorporate a GnRH analogue or GnRH antagonist and in which a fresh embryo transfer is planned.

LPS is used to offset the effect of the induced luteal phase insufficiency (the inability of the part of the ovary from which the eggs were collected to produce the hormones necessary to maintain a favorable uterine lining for implantation). This may cause embryo implantation to be compromised.

There is no demonstrable benefit if stimulation is accomplished with gonadotrophin (FSH) alone or in combination with clomiphene (a pill that tricks the brain into thinking estrogen levels are low and results in increased secretion of FSH, which stimulates follicular development and leads to ovulation), but without a GnRH agonist or GnRH antagonist.

In 2015, the most recent Cochrane Collaboration Systematic Review of Luteal Phase Support (LPS) confirmed that human Chorionic Gonadotrophin (hCG) injection, vaginal progesterone gel (Crinone), progesterone pessaries, and intramuscular injections of progesterone increased clinical and live birth rates, when compared to placebos (dummy medications) or no treatment.[1]

However, hCG LPS carries an increased risk of OHSS, especially if more than ten eggs are collected.

Intramuscular progesterone injections are not only painful, they can be complicated by infection and abscess formation at the injection site, and rarely, they even result in adult Respiratory Distress Syndrome (RDS) or eosinophilic pneumonia (a rare but very serious respiratory condition).

It has been demonstrated that vaginal progesterone pessary administration resulted in higher progesterone concentrations in endometrial (uterine lining) tissue than in the bloodstream.[2]

---

1   van der Linden M, Buckingham K, Farquhar C, Kremer JA, and Metwally M. *Luteal phase support for assisted reproduction cycles.* Cochrane Database Systematic Review. 2015.
2   Bulletti C, de Ziegler D, Flamigni C, Giacomucci E, Polli V, Bolelli G, and Franceschetti E. *Targeted drug delivery in gynaecology: the uterine first pass effect.* Hum. Reprod. 1997; 12:1073-1079.

The 2015 Cochrane Collaboration Systematic Review also found that the addition of a GnRH agonist to progesterone LPS significantly increased the live birth rate. It was unable to demonstrate that the addition of estradiol to LPS increased pregnancy rates.

However, a 2014 study did demonstrate a statistically significant improvement of the clinical pregnancy rate in poor responders (women who had less than four eggs collected in a stimulated cycle) when estradiol was added to progesterone LPS.[3]

A 2015 systematic review showed that there did not appear to be a difference whether LPS was started on the same day as the hCG trigger, egg collection, or cleavage (day two or three) embryo transfer.[4]

There is evidence from randomized controlled trials that progesterone supplements used for LPS can be withdrawn at the time of a positive pregnancy test without adverse effect (i.e. they do not need to be taken after positive pregnancy results).[5, 6]

3   Kutlusov F, Guler I, Erdem M, Erdem A, Bozkurt N, Biberoglu EH, and Biberoglu KO. *Luteal phase support with estrogen in addition to progesterone increases pregnancy rates in in vitro fertilization cycles with poor response to gonadotrophins.* Gynecol. Endocrinol. 2014; 30:363-366.

4   Connell MT, Szatkowski JM, Terry N, DeCherney A, Propst AM, and Hill MJ. *Timing luteal support in assisted reproductive technology: a systematic review.* Fertil. Steril. 2015; 103:939-946.

5   Kyrou D, Fatemi HM, Zepiridis L, Riva A, Papanikolaou EG, Tarlatzis BC, and DeVroey P. *Does cessation of progesterone supplementation during early pregnancy in patients treated with recFSH/GnRH antagonist affect ongoing pregnancy rates? A randomized controlled trial.* Hum. Reprod. 2011; 26:1020-1024.

6   Kohls G, Ruiz F, Martinez M, Hauzman E, de la Fuente G, Pellicer A, and Garcia-Velasco JA. *Early progesterone cessation after in vitro fertilization/intracytoplasmic sperm injection: a randomized controlled trial.* Fertil. Steril. 2012; 98:858-862..

❓ WHAT CAN I DO TO IMPROVE MY CHANCES OF CONCEPTION?

Vaginal progesterone is the Luteal Phase Support (LPS) of choice because it is not associated with the complications of intramuscular injections of progesterone and is equally effective. It also does not carry the risk of Ovarian Hyperstimulation Syndrome associated with the use of hCG for LPS.

The addition of a GnRH analogue to LPS in fresh embryo transfer cycles significantly increases the live birth rate.

CHAPTER 13

What Next?
Part 1:
Worth Considering

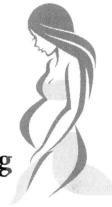

Options

If you have not successfully achieved a pregnancy, there are two main options: beginning another IVF cycle or ceasing IVF treatment altogether.

The first includes several different routes; you can continue to use your own eggs, or you can opt to use donor eggs, sperm, or embryos.

If you are considering beginning another treatment cycle using your own eggs, the options worth considering will depend on whether you are a normal responder, a poor responder (low ovarian reserve), or an over-responder (polycystic ovaries).

All of these paths will have some steps in common that may optimize outcomes, but each will have its own special requirements.

Hysteroscopy

Hysteroscopy (looking inside the uterine cavity with a very thin telescope passed through the cervical canal via the vagina) with endometrial biopsy (sampling of the uterine lining) and removal of any polyps or submucosal fibroids that have been identified with the assistance of saline contrast during a transvaginal ultrasound examination, should always be considered before further treatment.

The ultrasound examination may have also identified hydrosalpinges (blocked, fluid-filled fallopian tubes) that should be laparoscopically (using keyhole surgery) dealt with before beginning another IVF treatment cycle.

The endometrial biopsy tissue can be stained with CD 138 (a stain used specifically to identify a substance on the surface of plasma cells), which is currently the most accurate way of diagnosing chronic endometritis. If chronic endometritis is diagnosed, treatment with a two-week course of antibiotics should be followed by an endometrial biopsy as an office procedure to confirm its eradication.

Endometrial Scratching

In 2016, the United Kingdom's Royal College of Obstetricians and Gynaecologists, which has an international membership, stated in a Scientific Impact Paper that "The available evidence points towards a potential benefit of endometrial biopsy in women with recurrent implantation failure when performed in the cycle preceding the IVF treatment cycle."[1]

---

1   Royal College of Obstetricians and Gynaecologists. *Local Endometrial Trauma [Endometrial Scratch]: A Treatment Strategy to Improve Implantation Rates.* Scientific Impact Paper 2016; No 54.

Serum Progesterone on Day of hCG Trigger

If serum progesterone is greater than 1.5 ng/ml (5 nmol/L) on the day of the hCG trigger, the planned fresh embryo transfer should not be carried out and all embryos should be frozen for elective transfer in a subsequent natural or artificial cycle. Premature progesterone elevation can be responsible for the development of an unfavorable endometrium (uterine lining) for implantation because it is out of phase with the embryo's development (See Chapter 5, Is It My Lining).

Zona Selected Intracytoplasmic Sperm Injection (ICSI)

Zona selected ICSI involves seeing which sperm attach to an egg and using these for ICSI because they are believed to be the best quality sperm. This technique has been found to significantly improve clinical pregnancy rates in patients with poor outcomes in ICSI cycles. This was reported at the Annual Scientific Meeting of the Fertility Society of Australia in 2013.[2]

It had previously been reported that sperm binding to human zona pellucida (egg shell) is highly selective for double strand DNA (normal DNA). Sperm with single strand DNA or denatured DNA (both are abnormal types of DNA) bind less or do not bind at all to the zona pellucida, probably because of defects in motility (movement) and, more especially, morphology (formation).[3]

---

2   Sivendran K, Bourne H, and Liu AD. *Zona pellucida bound sperm for ICSI improves implantation and clinical pregnancy rate in couples with persistent poor outcomes in previous conventional cycles.* Fertility Society of Australia. 2013; Annual Scientific Meeting.
3   Liu DY and Baker HWG. *Human sperm bound to the zona pellucida have normal chromatin as assessed by acridine orange fluorescence.* Hum. Reprod. 2007; 22; 1597-1602.

Preimplantation Genetic Screening (PGS)

A chromosomally abnormal embryo, no matter how good its appearance or how well it develops, will not result in a normal ongoing pregnancy or delivery of a normal baby. Therefore, it makes sense that transferring only chromosomally normal embryos should result in better outcomes. This has been confirmed by numerous randomized controlled trials.

A 2013 study compared morphologically (structurally) based day five embryo transfers with day six transfers carried out after genetic testing. It showed a statistically significantly higher pregnancy rate in the group that underwent genetic testing.[4]

Another study, also carried out in 2013, concluded that cleavage stage (day three) embryo biopsy markedly reduced embryonic reproductive potential (the likelihood that the embryo would implant and continue growing) and that the blastocyst stage (day five) is the optimal time to perform an embryo biopsy for PGS.[5]

Stimulation Protocols

Normal Responders

According to a prospective randomized controlled study carried out in 2014, prolonged (28 day) pituitary down-regulation with a GnRH agonist statistically significantly improved implantation, clinical pregnancy, and live birth rates, when compared with the standard long down-regulated protocol (with a GnRH agonist

4   Scott RT, Upham KM, Forman EJ, Hong KH, Scott KL, Taylor D, Tao X, and Treff NR. *Blastocyst biopsy with comprehensive chromosome screening and fresh embryo transfer significantly increases in vitro fertilization implantation and delivery rates: a randomized controlled study.* Fertil. Steril. 2013; 100:697-703.
5   Scott KL, Hong KH, and Scott RT. *Selecting the optimal time to perform biopsy for preimplantation genetic testing.* Fertil. Steril. 2013;100:608-614.

started during the mid-luteal phase, day 21 of the cycle preceding the stimulation cycle).[6]

Simultaneous administration of 150 I.U. each of urinary Follicle Stimulating Hormone (uFSH) and recombinant Follicle Stimulating Hormone (recFSH) in a long down-regulated protocol with a 10,000 I.U. human Chorionic Gonadotrophin (hCG) trigger was used in a prospective randomized trial. It was compared with 300 I.U. of rec FSH and 300 I.U. of uFSH in patients who had at least three to five unsuccessful IVF stimulated cycles.

This 2013 study showed statistically significantly higher clinical pregnancy, implantation, and live birth rates in the protocol employing a combination of uFSH and rec FSH.[7]

Over-Responders

The safest option is a GnRH antagonist cycle with GnRH agonist triggering, and freezing all embryos for transfer in a subsequent natural or artificial cycle. This is not associated with a risk of Ovarian Hyperstimulation Syndrome.

Poor Responders

There is no proven value in increasing the daily dose of FSH above 300 I.U. In fact, there is no evidence-based protocol for poor responders.

However, multiple stimulated cycles using banking of frozen embryos could be considered to create enough embryos

---

6   Ren J, Sha A, Han D, Li P, Geng J, and Ma C. *Does prolonged pituitary down-regulation with gonadotropin-releasing hormone agonist improve the live-birth rate in in vitro fertilization treatment?* Fertil. Steril. 2014; 102:75-81.
7   Selman H, Pacchiarotti A, Rinaldi L, Crescenzi F, Lanzilotti G, Lofino S, and El-Danasouri I. *Simultaneous administration of human acidic and recombinant less acidic follicle-stimulating hormone for ovarian stimulation improves oocyte and embryo quality and clinical outcome in patients with repeated IVF failures.* Eur. Rev. Med. Pharmacol. Sci. 2013; 17:1814-1819.

to make PGS prior to embryo transfer both economically and emotionally viable.

Hyaluronic Acid (Hyaluronan, also known as EmbryoGlue)

The Cochrane Collaboration Collaboration updated its review of EmbryoGlue in 2014, analyzing 16 studies with a total of 3,898 participants. It concluded that "Evidence suggests improved clinical pregnancy and live birth rates with the use of functional (high as opposed to low) concentrations of hyaluronan as an adherence compound in ART (Artificial Reproduction Technology) cycles."[8]

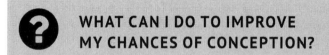

WHAT CAN I DO TO IMPROVE MY CHANCES OF CONCEPTION?

Before another embryo transfer is performed, hysteroscopy offers the opportunity to exclude previously undiagnosed submucosal fibroids or endometrial polyps. It also offers an opportunity for an endometrial biopsy to be performed to exclude chronic endometritis.

Blocked, fluid-filled fallopian tubes should be dealt with before any further embryo transfers.

Endometrial scratching (biopsy), which can be performed as an office procedure, increases the chances of implantation when there is a past history of recurrent implantation failure.

---

8   Bentekoe S, Heineman M, Johnson N, and Blake D. *Adherence compounds in embryo transfer media for assisted reproductive technologies.* Cochrane Collaboration Systematic Review. 2014.

Elevated serum progesterone on the day of the hCG trigger is an indication for freezing all embryos. In other words, performing a fresh embryo transfer is not recommended.

Zona selected ICSI involves seeing which sperm attach to an immature egg (one of the collected eggs that will not fertilize and will be discarded or used for research) and only using these sperm for microinjection. This creates the possibility of only using the best sperm for fertilization.

PGS does not increase the likelihood of a successful outcome per stimulated IVF cycle, but it does shorten the time to have a baby because chromosomally abnormal embryos, which are doomed to failure, are not being transferred.

Hyaluronan (EmbryoGlue) may be worth considering. It mimics natural uterine secretions that help with implantation.

CHAPTER 14

What Next?
Part 2:
Worth Discussing

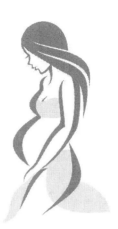

Melatonin

Melatonin is a very powerful antioxidant. It has been suggested that its antioxidative actions in follicular fluid may reduce the death of important cells and allow growing follicles to fully develop and provide mature (fertilizable) eggs for ovulation.

A 2008 study reported the effect of administering three milligrams of melatonin from day five of the previous cycle until egg collection in IVF treatment.[1]

Fifty-six subjects received the medication, while 59 were left untreated. The fertilization and pregnancy rates of the treated group were double those of the untreated group.

In 2014, a systematic review and meta-analysis of randomized controlled trials involving melatonin supplementation during ovarian stimulation for women undergoing assisted reproductive technology was performed. It came to the conclusion that more

---

1   Tamura H, Takasaki A, Miwa I, Taniguchi K, Maekawa R, Asada H, Taketani T, Maisuoka A, Yamagata Y, Shimamura K, Morioka H, Ishikawa H, Reiter RJ, and Sugino N. *Oxidative stress impairs oocyte quality and melatonin protects oocytes from free radical damage and improves fertilization.* J. Pineal Res. 2008; 44:280-287.

studies were still needed before recommending its use in clinical practice.[2] They did not include the Tamura study in the review because it had not been randomized.

Acupuncture

An evaluation of the evidence for complementary and alternative fertility treatments observed that "Although acupuncture may offer significant benefit, proof of its efficacy has been hampered by inadequate standardization of treatments."[3] Subsequently, in 2013, the Cochrane Collaborative Database Review concluded that "There is no evidence that acupuncture improves live birth and pregnancy rates."[4]

A very large, high quality prospective study, with randomized controls, is currently being conducted in Australia on the impact of acupuncture on IVF outcomes. The final results should be available by the end of 2017. This will hopefully provide a definitive answer.

Androgens and Androgen Modulating Drugs in Poor Responders

A systematic review and meta-analysis of this issue concluded that "Currently, based on available evidence, transdermal (applied to and absorbed through the skin) testosterone pre-treatment seems to increase clinical pregnancy and live birth rates in poor responders undergoing stimulation for IVF.

2   Seko LMD, Moroni RM, Leitao VMS, Teixeira DM, Nastri CO, and Martins WP. *Melatonin supplementation during controlled ovarian stimulation for women undergoing assisted reproductive technology: systematic review and meta-analysis of randomized controlled trials.* Fertil. Steril. 2014;101:154-161.

3   Weiss DA, Harris CR, and Smith JF. *The use of complementary and alternative fertility treatments.* Current Opinion Obstet. Gynecol. 2011; 23:195-199.

4   Cheong YC, Dix S, Hung Yu Ng E, Ledger WL, and Farquhar C. *Acupuncture and assisted reproductive technology.* Cochrane Collaboration Systematic Review. 2013.

There is insufficient evidence to support claims that recombinant Luteininizing Hormone (rLH), human Chorionic Gonadotrophin (hCG), dehydroepiandrosterone (DHEA), or letrozole administration play a beneficial role in the probability of pregnancy in poor responders undergoing ovarian stimulation for IVF."[5]

A review article, entitled "DHEA as a miracle drug in the treatment of poor responders: hype or hope?" came to the conclusion that "until well-designed large scale studies prove beyond reasonable doubt that DHEA improves ovarian reserve, its use should at best be considered experimental."[6]

Growth Hormone

The 2010 Cochrane Database review "demonstrated no difference in outcome measures and adverse events in routine use of adjuvant (improving the body's response) growth hormone in in vitro fertilization protocols."[7]

The authors did add, however, that "the use of growth hormone in poor responders had been found to show a significant improvement in live birth rates," but they "were unable to identify which sub-group of poor responders would benefit the most." They also said that "The results needed to be interpreted with caution (because) the included trials were few in number and small sample size."

---

5   Bosdou JK, Venetis CA, Kolibianakis EM, Toulis KA, Goulis DG, Zepiridis L, and Tarlatzis BC. *The use of androgens and androgen-modulating agents in poor responders undergoing in vitro fertilization: a systematic review and meta-analysis.* Hum. Reprod. Update 2012; 18:127-145.
6   Yakin K and Urman B. *DHEA as a miracle drug in the treatment of poor responders: hype or hope?* Hum. Reprod. 2011; 26:1941-1944.
7   Duffy JMN, Ahmad G, Mohiyiddeen L, Nardo LG, and Watson A. *Growth hormone for in vitro fertilization.* Cochrane Collaboration Systematic Review. 2010.

Dual Trigger

A 2013 study found that a dual trigger of final egg maturation (ripening) with Ovidrel (hCG) 6,500 I.U. and Lucrin (GnRH agonist) 0.2 mg in normal responders led to statistically significant improvement of implantation, clinical pregnancy, and live birth rates, versus a standard Ovidrel trigger alone.[8]

Fresh Versus Frozen Embryo Transfer

Not having a fresh transfer and instead freezing all embryos (and subsequently transferring a single thawed embryo in a natural or artificial cycle) eliminates the need to measure serum progesterone on the day of the hCG trigger. It also reduces concerns about Ovarian Hyperstimulation Syndrome (OHSS) and worries about the effect of ovarian stimulation on endometrial receptivity.

A 2013 systematic review and meta-analysis of the available literature on fresh versus frozen embryo transfer in IVF cycles summed it up like this: "results suggest that there is evidence that IVF outcomes may be improved by performing frozen embryo transfer compared with fresh embryo transfer."[9]

In 2014, a paper entitled "Clinical rationale for cryopreservation of entire embryo cohorts in lieu of fresh embryo transfer (i.e. freeze all, transfer later)" sensibly concluded that "although the trends have been steadily shifting in favor of cohort cryopreservation (freezing all embryos) and frozen embryo transfer on the basis of

8   Lin MH, Wu F S Y, Lee RK K, Li S H, Lin S Y, and Hwu Y M. *Dual trigger with combination of gonadotropin-releasing hormone agonist and human chorionic gonadotrophin significantly improves the live birth rate for normal responders in GnRH antagonist cycles.* Fertil. Steril. 2013; 100:1296-130.
9   Roque M, Lattes K, Serra S, Sola I, Geber S, Carreras R, and Checa MA. *Fresh embryo transfer versus frozen embryo transfer in in vitro fertilization cycles: a systematic review and meta-analysis.* Fertil. Steril. 2013; 99:156-162.

success results, there is not yet any clear choice that this maximizes success rates for all patients at all centers, and therefore individualized approaches remain appropriate."[10]

Endometrial Receptivity Assay (ERA)

The Endometrial Receptivity Assay identifies if a patient will require a personalized "window of implantation" before starting an IVF cycle.[11] The test claims to be able to evaluate a woman's endometrial receptivity (favorability of the uterine lining for implantation) from a molecular point of view.

Endometrial biopsy is carried out as an office procedure seven days after the LH surge. The specimen is analyzed for 238 genes related to endometrial receptivity. The result of this analysis determines if the patient was responsive to implantation at the time of the biopsy.

A state of non-receptivity means the window of implantation is displaced (moved), and the process will need to be repeated, according to data from the ERA predictor, which will give a new estimate of the personalized window of implantation. Once this is identified, the embryo may be successfully transferred in a subsequent cycle. The result is valid for at least three months.

10   Shapiro BS, Daneshmand ST, Garner FC, Aguirre M, and Hudson C. *Clinical rationale for cryopreservation of entire embryo cohorts in lieu of fresh embryo transfer.* Fertil. Steril. 2014; 102:3-9.
11   Ruiz-Alonso M, Blesa D, Diaz-Gimeno P, Gomez E, Fernandez-Sanchez M, Carranza F, Carrera J, Vitella F, Pellicer A, and Simon C. *The endometrial receptivity array for diagnosis and personalized embryo transfer as a treatment for patients with repeated implantation failure.* Fertil. Steril. 2013; 100:818-824.

Granulocyte Colony Stimulating Factor (G-CSF) Filgrastim (Neupogen)

A thin endometrial lining (equal to or less than seven millimeters) complicates 2.4% of IVF cycles, and it has been suggested that this compromises IVF success rates.[12]

There have been small observational studies, but no randomized prospective controlled studies, demonstrating that instilling G-CSF into the uterine cavity increases endometrial thickness.[13, 14]

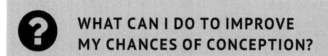

? WHAT CAN I DO TO IMPROVE MY CHANCES OF CONCEPTION?

Melatonin is a powerful antioxidant (a substance that protects cells, including possibly eggs, from being damaged). There will never be a high quality study of the potential benefits of melatonin in IVF because it is readily available, has no significant side effects, and is inexpensive. Persuading patients to be involved in a study where one half would receive a placebo (dummy medicine) and the other half would receive melatonin would be very difficult.

---

12   Kasius A, Smit JG, Torrance HL, Eijkemans MJ, Mol BW, Opmeer BC, and Broekmans FJ. *Endometrial thickness and pregnancy rates after IVF: a systematic review and meta-analysis.* Hum. Reprod. Update 2014; 20:530-541.
13   Kunicki M, Lukaszuk K, Woclawek-Potocka I, Liss J, Kulwikowska P, and Szczyptanska J. *Evaluation of Granulocyte Colony-Stimulating Factor Effects on Treatment-Resistant Thin Endometrium in Women Undergoing In Vitro Fertilization.* BioMed. Research International. 2014; Article ID 913235.
14   Lee D, Jo JD, Kim SK, Jee BC, and Kim SH. *The efficacy of intrauterine instillation of granulocyte colony-stimulating factor in infertile women with a thin endometrium: a pilot study.* Clin. Exp. Reprod. Med. 2016; 43:240-246.

Therefore, melatonin use warrants discussion with your fertility specialist.

A high quality Australia-wide acupuncture study should provide a definitive answer on its value for IVF outcomes by the end of 2017.

DHEA has significant side effects, and its value still needs to be proven.

Testosterone absorbed through the skin may benefit poor responders.

Dual triggering is a relatively new development in IVF treatment that may improve the percentage of mature eggs (capable of being fertilized) and hence may increase the number of embryos created.

The philosophy of freezing all embryos and not performing a fresh embryo transfer depends on the success of your IVF clinic's freezing program. What is the risk of losing a potentially perfectly normal embryo during the thawing process at your IVF clinic?

The use of Granulocyte Stimulating Factor (G-CSF), Filgastrim, warrants discussion if you have experienced recurrent implantation failure associated with a thin endometrium.

CHAPTER 15

What Next?

Part 3: Donor Eggs, Sperm, or Embryos

You realize that what you have been doing is not going to work, but your heart is still set on continuing. You still want to be a mother.

After considerable soul-searching, sessions with your IVF counselor, consultations with your fertility specialist, and discussions with those closest to you, you decide to proceed by finding a suitable donor.

Considerations for All Types of Donors

Whether you need donor eggs, sperm, or embryos, there are some questions that need to be answered. Most importantly, the donor's profile should be made available to you, including the following health information:

Q Past and family history of mental illness (e.g. schizophrenia)

Q Past and family history of inherited disease (e.g. spina bifida)

Q Results of screening tests for infectious diseases, including:

⚗ Hepatitis B

⚗ Hepatitis C

⚗ HIV

⚗ Syphilis

⚗ HTLV 1 (a virus implicated in several diseases, including lymphoma; in contrast, HTLV 2 has not been clearly linked to any disease)

Q Blood Group results and genetic testing for:

⚗ Thalassemia (inherited blood disorder that causes anemia and is most common among people of Greek, Italian, Middle Eastern, South Asian, and African descent)

⚗ Cystic fibrosis (inherited disorder that mainly affects the lungs and leads to a reduced life expectancy of less than 50 years. About 1 in 25 people is a carrier. Carriers have no symptoms, but the offspring of two carriers has a 1 in 4 chance of being affected by the condition)

⚗ Spinal-muscular atrophy (inherited disorder characterized by loss of nerves and muscle wasting, leading to an early death)

⚗ Fragile X (inherited disorder that is the most common cause of inherited intellectual disability; and 20% of women who are carriers have premature menopause, i.e. before the age of 40)

Sperm Donors

The age of sperm donors is important because DNA fragmentation increases with age, meaning that there is a reduced likelihood of a successful outcome. There is also an increased incidence of mental disorders and autism spectrum disorders with older sperm donors. It is always helpful to know the results of treatment cycles in which the donor's sperm has previously been used.

Egg Donors

An egg donor's age is critical to the outcome. She should be under 35. It would also be helpful to know the egg donor's ovarian reserve (assessed by measuring Anti-Mullerian Hormone levels and/or the Antral Follicle Count) because it would give an indication of how well she is going to respond to stimulation. This is discussed in detail in Chapter 1.

Knowing the outcomes of previous egg donations and her own pregnancies is essential when evaluating your egg donor.

Donor Embryos

For donor embryos, the age of the male partner at the time the embryos were created is important, but the age of the female partner in particular will have a significant impact on the likelihood of a successful outcome.

Another important factor to consider is at what stage of development the embryos were frozen. It is worth knowing if they were frozen at the cleavage stage (day two or day three) or the blastocyst stage (day five) because the latter have better prospects of achieving an ongoing pregnancy.

If they were frozen at the cleavage stage, the embryos could be thawed and allowed to grow to the blastocyst stage. Some embryos will not survive this journey, but those that do offer a better chance of pregnancy.

It is also helpful to know the history of the donor's embryos and their success rates. Have other embryos from this batch (embryos created from a single egg collection) resulted in pregnancies? Have embryos from another batch (from the same donor) resulted in pregnancies?

Receiving Donor Embryos

Embryo transfer should be performed under ultrasound control. You may wish to consider using EmbryoGlue (see Chapter 13).

Before further embryo transfers, you should seriously consider undergoing certain tests or procedures, if they have not been performed recently:

Q Ultrasound to exclude submucosal fibroids, endometrial polyps, and suspicion of adenomyosis

Q MRI to confirm adenomyosis, if suspected on ultrasound

Q Hysteroscopy to confirm ultrasound findings and endometrial biopsy to exclude chronic endometritis

Q Trial embryo transfer

Q Endometrial biopsy (endometrial scratching) the week before day one of the cycle in which the embryo will be transferred

The embryo transfer should not be carried out if there is fluid in the uterine cavity.

Single embryo transfer is advised with younger donors because there is a high risk of twins, triplets, and even quadruplets if two embryos are transferred because they could split during early development.

In Conclusion

I sincerely hope that this book has achieved its aim—to empower you with clear, factual information. Hopefully, this knowledge has enabled you to understand what has happened in the past and to plan for the best possible future outcome.

Good luck!

You deserve it.

Dr. Raphael Kuhn

Glossary

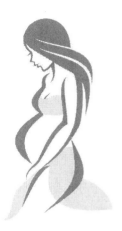

Acupuncture
The insertion of fine needles into the skin at specific points along what practitioners consider to be energy lines (meridians)

Adenomyosis
The abnormal presence of the endometrium (inner lining of uterus) within the myometrium (muscular wall of uterus)

Aneuploid
The presence of an abnormal number of chromosomes in a cell

Androgens
Hormones that influence the development and maintenance of male characteristics

Anti-Mullerian Hormone (AMH)
AMH is produced by the cells that line ovarian follicles awaiting further development.

Antiphospholipid Antibodies
The presence of these antibodies may indicate the presence of an acquired disorder that shows itself through recurrent venous or arterial thrombosis (clots).

Artificial Oocyte Activation
Manipulation to activate the sequence of processes that would normally occur in the egg after sperm entry/during fertilization

Body Mass Index (BMI)
Weight in pounds divided by height in inches squared x 703 or weight in kilograms divided by height in meters squared; used as a measure of health

Blastocyst
Formed about five days after fertilization, this consists of an inner cell mass (ICM), that later forms the fetus, an outer cell layer (called the trophoblast), that gives rise to the placenta and surrounds the ICM, and a fluid filled cavity, called the blastocele.

Clomiphene
A selective estrogen receptor modulator (SERM) that "tricks" the brain into thinking that estrogen levels are low, causing it to release the gonadotrophin Follicle Stimulating Hormone (FSH), which stimulates follicle development

Clinical Pregnancy Rate
The number of pregnancies (per 100 initiated cycles, aspiration cycles, or embryo transfer cycles) with a detectable fetal heartbeat or gestation sac; the denominator must be specified

Chromosome
A strand of DNA made up of genes; humans have 22 pairs of chromosomes plus 2 sex chromosomes (XX in female and XY in male), making a total of 46 chromosomes

Cleavage Stage Embryo
This refers to embryos two or three days post-fertilization. Their individual cells are called blastomeres. These then form a compact cell mass called the morula, which develops into a blastocyst by day five.

Cochrane Collaboration Systematic Review
Internationally recognized as a very high standard for evidence-based health care resources

DHEA
Dehydroepiandrostenedione, produced by the adrenal glands, gonads, and brain, is a precursor to androgen and estrogen sex hormones.

Endometrium
This is the lining of the uterus, the superficial part (lining the cavity) of which is shed with each period if pregnancy does not occur.

Endometrial Biopsy
A sample of uterine lining that can be obtained through hysteroscopy or as an office procedure

Endometrial Receptivity
Favorability of the uterine lining for embryo implantation

Endometriosis
Tissue that normally lines the uterus growing outside the uterus

Endometrioma
Benign, estrogen-dependent ovarian cyst lined with endometrial material and filled with clotted blood

Endometritis
Inflammation of the lining of the uterus

Euploid
Presence of a normal number of chromosomes in a cell

Fibroids
Benign uterine tumors made of smooth muscle and fibrous connective tissue

Follicle Stimulating Hormone (FSH)

FSH is produced by the pituitary gland and stimulates ovarian follicular growth, which results in the estrogen production responsible for the proliferation of the endometrium.

Germinal Vesicle (GV)

Large vesicular nucleus of an egg before meiotic division is completed, which results in the number of chromosomes in the parent cell being halved

Gonadotrophin

Refers to either FSH or LH

Gonadotrophin Releasing Hormone (GnRH)

A hormone released by the hypothalamus that acts on receptors in the pituitary gland and causes the release of FSH and LH.

Gonadotrophin Releasing Hormone agonist (GnRHa)

A synthetic hormone that mimics the effects of GnRH

Gonadotrophin Releasing Hormone antagonist (GnRH antagonist)

This blocks GnRH receptors and thus the action of GnRH, stopping the release of FSH and LH by the pituitary gland.

Growth Hormone

Hormone produced by the pituitary gland that stimulates the release of another hormone responsible for growth (Somatomedin) from the liver

Heparin

While primarily used as an anticoagulant (blood thinner), it also possesses anti-inflammatory and immunosuppressive properties.

human Chorionic Gonadotrophin (hCG)

Hormone produced by the placenta that maintains the corpus luteum during pregnancy; it is used to trigger final oocyte (egg) maturation in IVF/ICSI treatment cycles

Hydrosalpinx (plural: Hydrosalpinges)

Distally (far end) blocked fallopian tube filled with serous (clear) fluid

Hysteroscopy

Procedure that enables looking inside the uterine cavity via the vagina and cervical canal

Intracytoplasmic Sperm Injection (ICSI)

An In Vitro Fertilization (IVF) technique involving the introduction of an individual sperm cell into an individual egg cell

Implantation Rate

The number of gestation (pregnancy) sacs observed during an ultrasound examination, divided by the number of embryos transferred

Intramural

When used in connection with fibroids, this refers to their presence within the uterine wall.

Laparoscopy

Surgery involving only small incisions in the abdominal wall, often referred to as "keyhole surgery"

Live Birth Rate

This may be self-explanatory, but the denominator needs to be specified (i.e. per cycle started, per oocyte retrieval, or per embryo transfer).

Luteinizing Hormone (LH)

Hormone produced by the pituitary gland; a sharp rise triggers ovulation

Luteal Phase Support (LPS)

Administration of medication, usually progesterone, to support the function of the corpus luteum in IVF/ICSI cycles that involved the use of a GnRH agonist or GnRH antagonist because their use has compromised normal corpus luteum function (i.e. the maintenance of an endometrium favorable for embryo implantation)

Melatonin

Hormone produced by the pineal gland at the base of the brain that regulates the sleep-wake cycle and is also a powerful antioxidant

Natural Killer Cells

These are a type of white blood cell that are critical to the immune system.

Ovarian Reserve

Term used to describe the capacity of the ovaries to produce eggs that are capable of fertilization

Ovarian Hyperstimulation Syndrome (OHSS)

An overreaction to controlled ovarian hyperstimulation; this only occurs if hCG is used as an ovulation trigger or for luteal support when an abnormally large number of follicles has developed during stimulation.

Oxidative Stress

Imbalance between production of free radicals and antioxidant defenses (i.e. more free radicals than antioxidants)

Progesterone

Hormone produced by the corpus luteum that stimulates the uterine lining to prepare for pregnancy

Pronucleus (plural: pronuclei)

The nucleus of a sperm or an egg during fertilization (after sperm entry into the egg, but before they fuse)

Recombinant Hormones

These are genetically engineered and replace the need for human-derived (usually urinary) equivalents (e.g. rec FSH, rec LH, and rec hCG).

Submucosal

When applied to fibroids, this refers to ones that are protruding into the uterine cavity.

Subserosal

When applied to fibroids, this refers to their presence on the surface of the uterus.

Zona Pellucida

Thick, transparent membrane surrounding an oocyte (egg)

Zygote

Fertilized egg with 46 chromosomes; this results from the fusion of the male and female pronuclei, which have 23 chromosomes each

Acknowledgements

After being rejected by mainstream publishers, who indicated there would be no readers for this type of book, it was Julie Postance of *iinspire media* who persuaded me to self-publish.

As a book publishing consultant, Julie not only guided me through writing this book, but also putting it together (i.e. cover design, editing, typesetting, social media content, and marketing.) I cannot adequately express my gratitude to her.

Creating an appealing front cover was challenging, but 99designs provided many interesting submissions, of which the Halder Group's proposal proved to be the favorite.

Jessica Higgins, Upwork, was a sensitive, down-to-earth, and insightful editor, who helped to create a more reader-friendly text.

Sandra Dill, CEO of ACCESS Australia, read the manuscript and made the type of helpful comments that must be incorporated into any book encompassing these issues.

Juliet Robinson, Chairperson of Melbourne IVF Human Ethics and Research Committee, carefully studied the content and made the book even more accessible.

Suresh Nair, IVF specialist, reviewed the manuscript and reinforced my feelings that this was information that needed to be made available to every IVF patient and clinician in order to make their journey together a more successful one. His support has been invaluable.

Koen Geerinckx, fertility specialist, upon reading the manuscript, was quick to point out that the information provided was also relevant to anyone about to begin IVF treatment so that they minimized the risk of failure.

Ian Rose, patent and copyright lawyer, provided a very reassuring opinion that, in this type of book, short quotations with appropriate acknowledgement of their source were within the spirit of the Copyright Act.

Marianne Tome, IVF counselor, looked at the book from a different perspective. She highlighted the importance of IVF counselors in supporting patients so that they do not abandon treatment prematurely when disappointment can otherwise become overwhelming.

Nelly Murariu, graphic designer, PixBee Design, who was responsible for the layout of the book, greatly enhanced the appeal of the front and back covers, and was an outstanding asset to the project.

My son, Sabien, an IT and strategic marketing expert, gently helped me get my "learner's permit" in the world of social media and IT.

Caroline, my wife, showed incredible patience over the course of this year-long project as I disappeared into my study updating and rewriting my ever-changing manuscript.

No one could have done it alone.

Thank you all.

You made it possible.

Hopefully, it will make a difference.

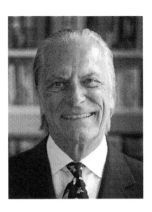

About the Author

Dr Raphael Kuhn was Senior Lecturer in the Department of Obstetrics and Gynaecology at The University of Melbourne, and later Head of the Gynaecology Department at both The Royal Melbourne Hospital and The Royal Women's Hospital. He spent more than 15 years as a consultant at Melbourne IVF and four years as Chairman of Melbourne IVF Human Research and Ethics Committee. In 2015, he created Infertility Second Opinion and spent two years providing independent opinions to patients who had not experienced IVF success.

The cases he saw during those two years prompted him to write this book.

Raphael is also a member of the Fertility Society of Australia (FSA), European Society of Human Reproduction and Embryology (ESHRE), and American Society for Reproductive Medicine (ASRM).

On a more personal note, his empathy for the issues addressed in this book stem from personal family experiences on the emotional roller coaster associated with IVF treatment.

66027967R00071

Made in the USA
Middletown, DE
07 March 2018